TECHNICAL MANUAL OF ANESTHESIOLOGY
An Introduction

Technical Manual of Anesthesiology
An Introduction

James E. Heavner, D.V.M., Ph.D.
Professor, Anesthesiology and Physiology
Director of Anesthesia Research
Associate Director, Anesthesia OR
Special Functions Laboratory
Texas Tech University Health Sciences Center
Lubbock, Texas

Craig Flinders
3rd Year Medical Student, Texas Tech University School of Medicine
Former Chief Anesthesia Technician
Texas Tech University Health Sciences Center, LGH
Lubbock, Texas
Former Anesthesia Technician
University of Utah School of Medicine
Salt Lake City, Utah

Dennis J. McMahon, B.S., C.B.E.T.
Chief Anesthesia Technician
Virginia Mason Clinic
Seattle, Washington

Tim Branigan, B.S.
Chief Anesthesia Technician
University of Utah School of Medicine
Salt Lake City, Utah

J. Michael Badgwell, M.D.
Assistant Professor, Anesthesiology and Pediatrics
Head, Pediatric Anesthesia
Medical Director, Anesthesia Technicians
Texas Tech University Health Sciences Center
Lubbock, Texas

Raven Press   New York

Raven Press, 1185 Avenue of the Americas, New York, New York 10036

Made in the United States of America

International Standard Book Number 0-88167-515-6

Library of Congress Cataloging-in-Publication Data

Technical manual of anesthesiology : an introduction / James E.
    Heavner . . . [et al.].
        p.   cm.
    Bibliography: p. 158
    Includes index.
    ISBN 0-88167-515-6
    1. Anesthesiology. I. Heavner, James. E.
    [DNLM: 1. Anesthesia. 2. Anesthesiology. WO 200 T255]
    RD81.T43 1989
    617.9′6—dc20
    DNLM/DLC
    for Library of Congress   89-8374
                                                               CIP

The material contained in this volume was submitted as previously unpublished material, except in the instances in which credit has been given to the source from which some of the illustrative material was derived.

Great care has been taken to maintain the accuracy of the information contained in the volume. However, neither Raven Press nor the editors can be held responsible for errors or for any consequences arising from the use of the information contained herein.

9 8 7 6 5 4 3 2 1

Foreword

Anesthesia is becoming safer and its quality is improving. This is reflected in the gradual shift of anesthesiology in the malpractice ratings from the highest risk group to an increasingly lower risk category. Credit for this goes to improved quality of staff in anesthesiology as well as new technology that renders the patient's visit to the operating room much safer. Anesthetic mortality remains in the range of 1 in 10,000 but with the present trend I am convinced that this ratio will be reduced. The increasing sophistication of the operating room has resulted in increased patient safety, and as a result, the field of anesthesiology has earned greater respect among other medical specialists, particularly surgeons. Conflicts in the operating room setting are becoming rarer and more emphasis is placed on prior consultation, discussion, and planning of the anesthetic.

Invasive monitoring must be available to every patient who enters the operating room. Staff caring for patients in the operating room require the same information needed by those in the intensive care setting. New technology has increased safety for operating room personnel by the use of scavenging techniques to prevent the environmental pollution that affects not only the patient but also all personnel present in the operating room. Basic monitors available in every operating room may include disconnect alarms, oxygen monitors, pulse oximeters, capnometers, mass spectometers, evoke potentials, respiratory gas monitors, and ventilation monitors. The American Society of Anesthesiologists has standards for the practice of anesthesia that require rigorous monitoring, including the use of electrocardiographic monitors, pulse oximeters, and capnometers.

The cost of this equipment has grown increasingly in the last few years. The cost also is growing in not only the initial purchase but to stretch the precious health care dollars by keeping the life of the equipment in safe and functional state of readiness at all times. Therein lies the need for personnel who understand all the equipment and who can operate it efficiently. A new type of individual thus is emerging in the form of the anesthesia technician, who must be familiar with all the equipment available to the anesthesia care team. Maintenance schedules must be meticulously observed so that possible faults are detected before they could jeopardize a patient's life.

Another area where sophisticated technical support is required by anesthesiologists is STAT lab determinations, particularly in tertiary care level insitutions, where it is quite common to have within the operating room an anesthesia laboratory run by the department of anesthesiology. It is typical to have automated equipment that will measure blood gases, blood sugars, oxygen saturation, electrolytes, osmolalities, urine, proteins, clotting profiles, and whatever the particular institution is specializing in where information must be available in a very brief period of time. These laboratory facilities must be accredited by appropriate agencies such as the College of American Pathologists or the JCAH (Joint Commission for the Accreditation of Hospitals). Accreditation is possible regardless of who runs these labs. The anesthesia technician therefore must be able to interact with the anesthesia personnel, the hospital administration, the accreditating agencies, and the vendors and manufacturers who are always developing newer and more sophisticated equipment. The choice of equipment must be made not only on the basis of equipment quality on the day of purchase but also the availability and need for service, and the availability and cost of maintenance agreements, as well as the reputation of the manufacturers.

Given these increased technical demands, it is no longer appropriate to place the available operating room orderly in charge of anesthesia equipment. Nevertheless, education requirements have not yet been specified for anesthesia technicians. Often it has been left to the initiative of the individual hired to take care of the anesthesia equipment. Readily available explicatory text has been sadly lacking and often the anesthesia technician may not have the background experience required to review individual manufacturer pamphlets and large textbooks. This book attempts to help fill the educational void for all anesthesia personnel.

Clearly there is a need for organized training and an examination system for all personnel involved in the preparation of the anesthesic site for maximum patient safety. It is hoped that this need will be recognized initially in community colleges or other major universities, and that an accreditated educational system will be developed in the next few years.

This introductory text is an important contribution to patient safety in the operating room. Therefore, the material should be utilized by nurses, doctors, and medical students, as well as the principal group of equipment users, the anesthesia technicians. This manual is a collection of relevant information for all anesthesia personnel.

Gabor Racz, M.D.
Professor and Chairman
Department of Anesthesiology
Texas Tech University
Health Sciences Center
Lubbock, Texas

Contents

Chapter 1

Introduction

Administration of an anesthetic involves a series of tasks that vary in complexity and in degree of skill required for their successful execution. Many of the tasks *can* be performed by non-anesthesiologists/non-anesthetists, although for various reasons, the anesthesiologist[1]/anesthetist[2] may do them. Our aim in this book is to present in a generally comprehensive manner discussion of those tasks. Emphasis will be placed on tasks that require some degree of skill and require rendering some judgment. The reader is referred to *The Anesthesia Care Team,* a pamphlet that discusses delegation of tasks, published by the American Society of Anesthesiologists (ASA).

As anesthesiologists/anesthetists use a wide variety of equipment, many of the tasks described in this book are associated with the use of this equipment. In broad terms, these tasks include setting-up and calibrating equipment prior to use, operating the equipment, taking appropriate action if malfunctions occur while in use, and maintaining the equipment.

Other tasks include those related to preparing the anesthetizing location (stocking drugs and supplies, etc.), assisting with patient preparation (applying monitoring sensors, positioning, etc.), running tests (blood gas analysis, etc.), and assisting with the immediate postoperative management of patients.

Anesthetic techniques can be separated into two groups: those involving general anesthesia and those involving regional anesthesia. General anesthesia renders a patient totally unconscious, whereas patients given regional anesthesia are at least partially awake. Supplies and equipment

---

[1]An *anesthesiologist* is an M.D. or D.O. who has completed residency training in anesthesiology.

[2]In the United States an *anesthetist* is usually an RN who has completed specialized training in anesthesiology; in other countries (e.g., Canada, Great Britain) an anesthetist is an MD who has completed residency training.

In this book anesthesiologist and anesthetist will be used, unless otherwise indicated, to designate the person administering the anesthetic.

used for general and regional anesthesia vary although there are some common elements.

The anesthesia machine and/or a constant infusion device are the primary devices used to administer general anesthetics. Breathing of anesthetized patients usually is controlled with ventilators (stand alone or part of the anesthetic machine). Specialized needles and catheters as well as syringes are the primary devices used to administer regional anesthesia.

According to standards approved by the ASA, the patient's oxygenation, ventilation, circulation, and temperature will be continuously evaluated during anesthesia.

It is *very* important to realize that operating room personnel are exposed to a number of personal health related risks. Particularly notable risks include exposure to AIDS and to hepatitis, and to anesthetic vapors. Hospitals generally have standard operating procedures and guidelines to follow to minimize these risks. All operating room personnel should be familiar with the procedures and adhere to them.

In order to understand the scope of responsibilities that an anesthesiologist might assign to a technical assistant (anesthesia technician), we begin by describing the set-up of an operating room for anesthesia care (Fig. 1).

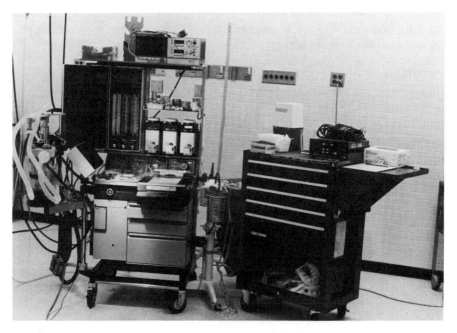

FIG. 1. OR set up and ready for patient. Anesthetic machine (**left**) and supply cabinet (**right**) are ready for case to start.

THE ANESTHESIA SET-UP

This discussion describes the anesthetic set-up procedure for surgical cases, giving particular attention to specialized equipment and supplies the anesthesiologist may need to provide safe regional or general anesthesia. It should be understood that there are some equipment and supplies that must be present and readily available to the anesthesiologist in all cases, regional or general. In many clinical situations there is pressure to keep to a minimum the time between surgical cases (turnover time). In these situations, cleaning equipment, setting up new equipment, and bringing in new supplies become the responsibility of someone other than the person administering the anesthetic. During much of this time the anesthesiologist is busy transporting and stabilizing the previous patient as well as reviewing the chart and preparing the next patient.

Routine General Anesthesia

This set-up procedure and the following routine need to be performed before any anesthetic procedure in the operating room begins.

1. Turnover room after previous case. This includes discarding all used, disposable items, cleaning anesthesia machine and monitors with disinfectant, washing laryngoscope blade and handle as described in Chapter 4, and discarding drugs according to the request of the anesthesiologist.
2. Place new breathing circuit, check CO_2 absorber and change if necessary, perform low pressure check on anesthetic machine (as described in Chapter 3), check ventilator function according to procedure, calibrate O_2 monitor, place new temperature probe, inspect and clean ECG cable and leadwires, verify electrical supply to machine and all monitors.
3. Lay out disposable items to be used: oral airway, tongue depressor, breathing mask (may or may not be disposable), endotracheal tubes, esophageal stethoscope, ECG electrodes, peripheral nerve stimulator electrodes, heat and moisture exchanger, alcohol swabs, IV catheters, gauge 4 × 4's, IV solution and tubing.
4. Place new suction canister, tubing, and tip, and verify functioning suction.
5. Check presence and function of laryngoscopes, replace batteries in handle if light is dim, or replace bulb if necessary.
6. Check peripheral nerve stimulator. Touch prongs or leads to thenar eminence (the mound on the thumb at the base of the thumb), place in pulse mode, turn dial to mid-range and gradually increase to maximum (if weak replace batteries; some models give light signal with decreased battery strength).

7. Place hypo/hyperthermia blanket on OR table, adjust setting, and turn on.
8. Place head rest, ulnar nerve protectors, arm straps on the OR table.
9. Make sure routine drugs are readily available to anesthesiologist.
10. Check blood pressure cuff and/or other blood pressure monitoring equipment, and verify proper functioning.

The anesthesiologist should discuss any special set-ups (i.e., transducers for invasive monitoring, EEG monitoring, special catheters or kits, etc.) with the technician prior to the patient being brought into the OR, thus allowing time for equipment and supplies to be gathered, assembled, arranged and/or calibrated. Good communication between the anesthesiologist and technical staff enhances efficient performance in the operating room and helps to ensure optimal care for the surgical patient.

THE ANESTHESIA TECHNICIAN

We and other interested parties have attempted through surveys, as well as informal and formal discussions, to determine who provides technical assistance to anesthesiologists in the United States and to obtain information about these people. Every question yielded a heterogeneous response—salaries range from minimum wage to more than $30,000/year; training ranges from on-the-job to completion of formal training programs; educational background ranges from high school graduates to PhD's, etc. Many respondents express a need for recognition at the national level of the anesthesia technician, in addition to definition of minimum qualifications, job description, and career ladder.

Chapter 2

Patient Positioning

The role of the anesthesia technician in positioning the patient usually is to provide place supports and pads, and to assist in moving the patient.

"Existing literature describing the requirements, techniques and consequences of positioning a patient for surgery is sparse, widely scattered and difficult to assemble. It is easy to overlook, but is of vital importance to all members of the anesthesia and surgical teams. Not uncommonly proper selection of patient posture during surgery affects the surgeon's access to the pathology as well as the patient's tolerance to anesthetic drugs and physical stresses. Thus, a clear understanding of the subject should be available to each participant if a cooperative venture such as an efficient surgical operation is to succeed."

This quotation from the preface of the First Edition of *Positioning in Anesthesia and Surgery* by J. T. Martin provides a good introduction to the subject of patient positioning. The Second Edition of Dr. Martin's book is the most recent, authoritative, and comprehensive discussion of the subject. In this section, we present a survey of the topic and refer the reader to *Positioning in Anesthesia and Surgery* for more detailed information.

First we will discuss the different positions used and special equipment requirements, and then describe complications of positioning. Chapter titles of Dr. Martin's book suggest that the identifiable and relatively common positions include: (1) the traditional supine position, (2) the prone position, and (3) the lawn chair (contoured supine) position, (4) the Trendelenburg position, (5) the lateral decubitus position, (6) the lithotomy position, (7) the head elevated position, and (8) unusual positions for orthopedic and urological procedures (Fig. 1). All positions originate from three basic ones—prone, supine, or lateral recumbency.

Various types of operating tables are available, including the general operating table, an orthopedic table, and a urology table. The general operating table, which is adjustable for height, is most commonly used. The top of the general operating table is usually divided into four parts: head, back, thighs, and feet (Fig. 2A). A fifth section, the kidney rest, is located between the back and thigh sections. Adjustment of the various

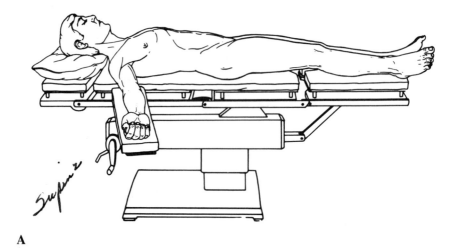

A

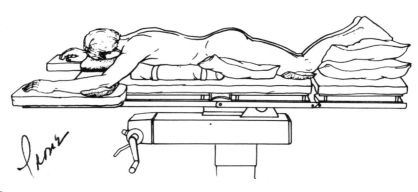

B

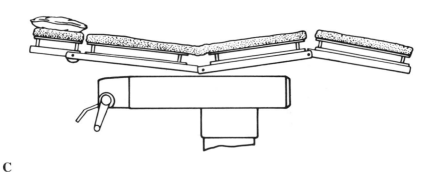

C

FIG. 1. Relatively common surgical positions: (**A**) supine, (**B**) prone, (**C**) surgical table in lawn chair (contoured supine) position. (*Figure continues.*)

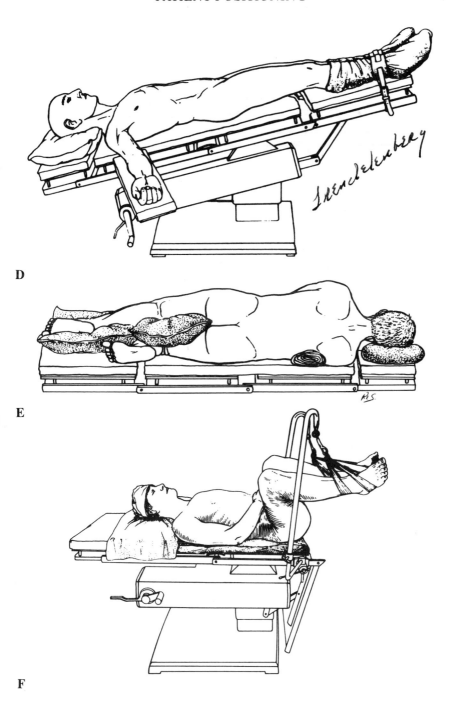

FIG. 1 (*Continued*). (**D**) Trendelenberg, (**E**) right lateral decubitus, (**F**) lithotomy. (*Figure continues.*)

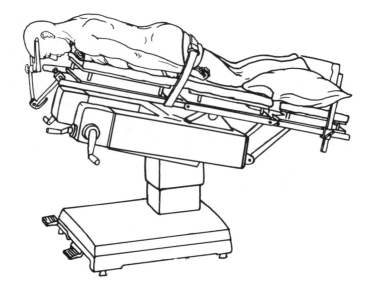

G

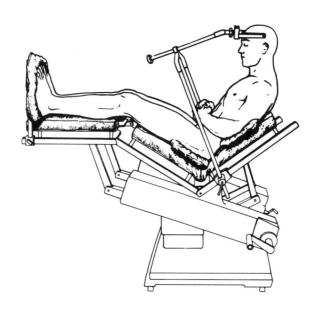

H

FIG. 1 (*Continued*).   (**G,H**) head elevated. (Reprinted with permission from J. T. Martin (ed) (1987): *Positioning in Anesthesia and Surgery,* 2nd ed. W. B. Saunders Co. Philadelphia, PA.)

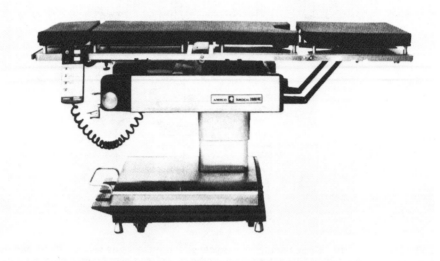

A

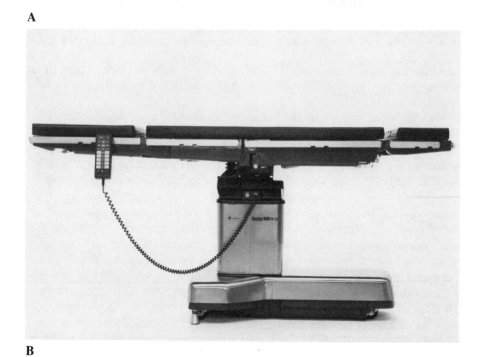

B

FIG. 2. A. Manually controlled surgical operating table. **B.** Remotely controlled table. (Courtesy of American Sterilizer Company.) (*Figure continues.*)

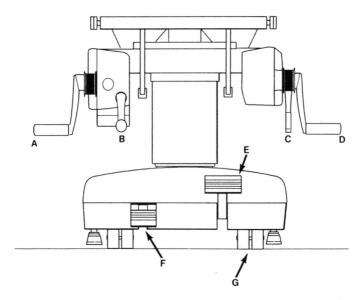

FIG. 2 (*Continued*).   **C.** Schematic of surgical operating table as viewed from head of table showing position of levers for adjusting the table. (A) Lever controlling horizontal tilt of the table, (B) lever controlling elevation of the kidney rest, (C) multiselector bar for activating foot, lateral (side-to-side) rotation, back and flex of the table, (D) lever regulating range of movement of multiselector bar, (E) foot-operated lever for table elevation, (F) floor lock, (G) wheels. (Reproduced with permission from R. M. Julien (1984): *Understanding Anesthesia.* Addison-Wesley Publishing Co., Menlo Park, CA.)

sections are made using levers (Fig. 2B) or a remote control unit. The kidney rest is sometimes disabled as it is considered by some physicians to be dangerous.

Various attachments to the table are available, e.g., arm board (Fig. 1A), supports for the "anesthesia screen" (Figs. 3A,B), bars for the lithotomy position (Fig. 1F), various supporting bars for neurosurgical procedures (Figs. 1G,H), and various bars for orthopedic procedures (Fig. 4). The tables are also equipped with straps for holding the patient in position.

Lateral table edges should be padded to prevent compression of nerves, vessels, tendons, and other vital structures. It is common for ulnar nerve protector pads to be used on all patients and for axillary rolls to be used when patients are in the lateral position. Head cradles and "donuts" help to ensure a safe and comfortable position. Many companies manufacture positioning pads and supports that will accommodate all sizes of patients, in many positions. Body parts should be protected from table hinges and restraining straps must be clean, intact, and positioned so damage to underlying bony prominences or neurovascular bundles will not occur. Monitoring lines and vascular lines should be kept clear of adjustment levers and table hinges.

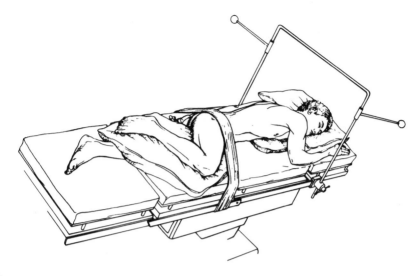

A

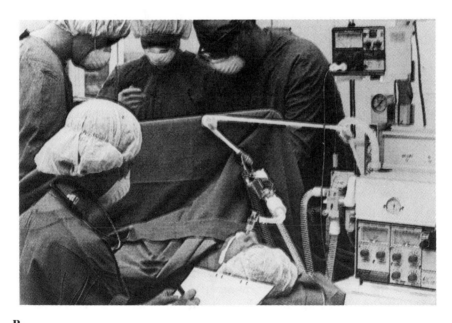

B
FIG. 3. **A.** Bar for anesthesia screen. (Reprinted with permission from J. T. Martin (ed) (1987): *Positioning in Anesthesia and Surgery,* 2nd ed. W. B. Saunders Co. Philadelphia, PA.) **B.** Ether screen in place. (Courtesy of Siemens-Elema Company.)

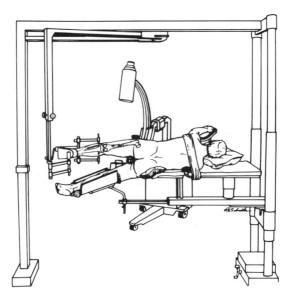

FIG. 4. Schematic of positioning equipment for an orthopedic procedure. (Reprinted with permission from J. T. Martin (ed) (1987): *Positioning in Anesthesia and Surgery,* 2nd ed. W. B. Saunders Co. Philadelphia, PA.)

A host of complications related to positioning have been reported. *Positioning in Anesthesia and Surgery* devotes one chapter to central nervous system (CNS) complications and another to peripheral nervous system (PNS) complications. Causes of these complications include, but are not limited to, pressure on nerves, stretching of nerves, and failure to control movement in patients with cervical instability. Amputation or injury to body parts trapped in hinges of the operating table may occur. Localized pressure damage may occur and ischemic injury secondary to vascular occlusion via pressure can occur.

Unusual patients, according to Martin, include pediatric, obstetrical, and pathologically obese patients. Two key factors related to positioning of pediatric patients are the large size of the head and the ease with which body temperature can be lost. It is necessary, because of the large head size, to protect the ears from pressure damage if the child is to be on one side for any period of time. A number of factors predispose pediatric patients to heat loss, including the fact that the operative site frequently necessitates total, or nearly total, exposure of the child. The most common positioning requirement in the obstetrical patient is left lateral displacement of the uterus. If the uterus is not displaced it may compress the vena cava, which in turn produces hypotension via reduced venous return. Positioning of morbidly obese patients is primarily a matter of scale (e.g., two operating tables may be required), and of the need for awareness by the anesthesiologists that physiological changes associated with different positions may be exaggerated in the obese patient. Also it is important to consider as unusual patients who, for one reason or another, cannot be positioned exactly as desired. Examples of such patients are those with fused joints (e.g., vertebrae, knees). It is essential that patients are checked before being anesthetized to be sure that they can be positioned as planned.

Chapter 3

The Anesthesia Machine

The anesthesia machine is used to deliver oxygen and other gases as well as anesthetic agents to the patient. An anesthetic machine ready for use is shown in Chapter 1, Figure 1. There are a variety of different machines produced by different manufacturers, but the basic design of the continuous flow anesthesia machine is essentially the same as the first closed-circuit system built more than 70 years ago. Many additional components have been integrated since to increase efficiency, reliability, and safety of the system. Over the years significant hazardous features of anesthesia machines have been realized and in an effort to eliminate these, the American National Standards Committee Z79, composed of engineers, nurses, and anesthesiologists produced the American National Standard Institute (ANSI) Z79.8, 1979, "Minimum Performance and Safety Requirements for Components and Systems of Continuous-Flow Anesthesia Machines for Human Use." (The American Society for Testing Materials (ASTM) F-29 committee is now responsible for this function). All anesthesia machines sold in the United States after 1983 are required to comply with these standards. Additionally, regulations under the Medical Device Amendments of 1976 (PL-94-295) give authority to the Food and Drug Administration (FDA) to regulate medical equipment for efficiency and safety. Distributors and manufacturers of medical equipment must report to the FDA within 5 days by telephone and within 15 days in writing the following: any equipment or device that has caused death or serious injury, any malfunction that could cause death or injury, any inaccurate information that may lead to improper usage or treatment, and remedial action taken by the manufacturer. The anesthetist can also report equipment problems directly to the FDA. The reliability of anesthesia machines is extremely high as a result of these actions and standards, and is further assured by preventive maintenance performed on a regular basis by qualified personnel. However, it is important to keep in mind that few things are perfect and occasionally equipment fails, and thus it is imperative that the operator and support personnel be knowledgeable about the various components and their function and interaction in the anesthesia machine. It has been well-documented that a significant number of preventable anesthetic mishaps are a result of human error due to inadequate experience or lack of familiarity with the anesthetic apparatus.

This chapter on the anesthesia machine is intended to provide the basis for an understanding of the workings of a simple anesthesia machine and its corresponding components, as well as how to check and determine its proper function. For a much more in-depth look at these aspects, the reader is encouraged to consult the sources in the Bibliography.

GAS FLOW THROUGH TWO-GAS ANESTHESIA MACHINE

Figure 1 illustrates gas flow and mixing as well as functional components encountered in a typical two-gas anesthesia machine. On examining the gas flow through the machine, one must realize that oxygen and nitrous oxide may be supplied from either the wall supply or from cyl-

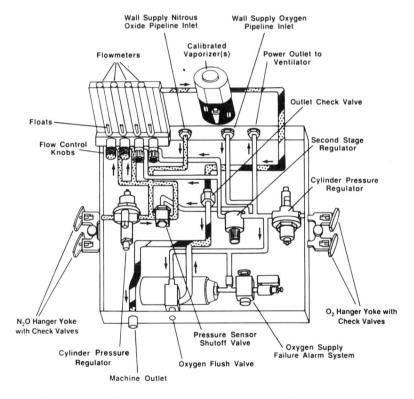

FIG. 1. Routes of gas flow and mixing as well as functional components encountered in a typical two-gas machine. ▒▒▒ indicates N_2O, ═══ indicates O_2, and ▄▀ indicates volatile inhalation agent. Arrows indicate direction of gas flow. (Reprinted with permission of Ohmeda, 1985. The BOC Group, Inc., Madison, WI.)

inders through the hanger yoke assembly (see Chapter 9). The gas then travels through pressure reducing valves to the flow control knobs where flow is controlled through the flowmeters. The gases mix with each other after ascending the flowmeters and pass through the calibrated vaporizer, where anesthetic agent is added to the mixture. The gas mixture then exits the machine via the machine outlet to enter the patient circuit.

THE FUNCTION OF THE MAJOR COMPONENTS

Wall Versus Cylinder Supply of Gases

Gas to the machine may be supplied from either the wall supply (the built-in gas system within the hospital) or the cylinders attached to the hanger yoke assembly. Wall supply pressure is typically 50 psi, a full cylinder of oxygen is 2,200 psi and nitrous oxide is 750 psi. Therefore, distal to the hanger yoke assembly is a cylinder pressure regulator that reduces the pressure from the cylinder to that of the wall source (40 to 60 psi). The double yoke assembly (Fig. 1) allows two cylinders of the same gas to be mounted to the anesthesia machine. Usually the cylinders are used only as a backup to the wall supply or if the machine is used when there is no piped-in gas. In this double yoke system, the gauge will indicate the pressure in the fullest tank when both cylinders are turned on. Therefore, each tank must be tested separately to be certain that each is full. There is a check valve inside each yoke assembly which eliminates the possibility of the cylinder of higher pressure emptying into the lower one (when both tanks are opened). There is also a check valve at the wall supply pipeline inlet which blocks gas flow from the machine into the wall supply when cylinders are being used as a gas source. When a cylinder position is unoccupied, a block supplied by the manufacturer should be in place to eliminate the possible leakage of gas. It is recommended that when using cylinders as the gas supply, only one cylinder be turned on at a time in a double-yoke assembly, thereby providing the assurance of always having a full cylinder available. When using the wall supply as the source of gas, one must be certain to remember to keep all cylinders closed. If the cylinder pressure regulator is set to reduce the pressure to something higher than the wall supply, then the check valve in the wall supply pipeline inlet will close. If this occurs the cylinders will be the only source of gas and they may become depleted without the user's knowledge.

Power Outlet to Ventilator

This pathway provides a means of supplying pneumatic power to a ventilator. There is a valve that remains closed unless the proper connector is attached, thereby depressing the valve off its seat and allowing oxygen to flow into the pneumatics of the ventilator. One must be sure to understand that this oxygen never enters the ventilator bellows or patient circuit, it only provides a pneumatic source to drive the ventilator. The oxygen flow required by the pneumatics of the ventilator may be considerable; therefore, when using the cylinders as the oxygen source, the cylinders may become depleted sooner than expected.

Oxygen Supply Failure Alarm and the Pressure Sensor Shutoff Valve (Fail-Safe Devices)

These devices are both safety components designed to warn the user of a drop in oxygen pressure and to protect the patient from a hypoxic mixture of gases when oxygen pressure is lost. The oxygen supply failure alarm is a pressure sensitive device designed to produce a loud audible alarm (usually a whistle) whenever the oxygen pressure drops below 50% of normal. When the machine is in use and the oxygen pressure is lost, the alarm should sound for at least 7 seconds, thus providing time for the user to either turn on the backup cylinder or change to a full one. In Figure 1 this device is located upstream of the second stage regulator and therefore alarms when the oxygen pressure reaches 20 to 30 psi (depending on the manufacturer). Once the oxygen pressure has been elevated above the alarm setting, the noise should cease. The user must realize that this alarm is not activated when pressure of any gas other than oxygen is lost; therefore, the oxygen concentration in the fresh gas flow may change without warning to the anesthetist.

The pressure sensor shutoff valve is also referred to by a variety of other names: Fail Safe, Oxygen Failure Safety Valve, and Oxygen Supply Pressure Failure Device (Fig. 2). This device, as the name implies, is sensitive to oxygen pressure within the anesthesia machine and is required by the ANSI machine standard. The function of this valve is to stop the flow of all gases other than oxygen whenever the oxygen supply pressure drops below 50% of normal. Usually the oxygen failure alarm is set slightly above the pressure sensor shutoff valve, thus the user is alerted before the drop in gas flow actually occurs. The user should understand that these safety devices are limited in their ability to protect the patient from a hypoxic mixture of gas; therefore, an oxygen analyzer should always be used in the patient circuit.

The Oxygen Flush Valve

When this valve is depressed, oxygen flows at a high rate (35 to 75 lpm) directly into the common gas line near the machine outlet (Fig. 1). It is used to rapidly fill the patient circuit. This flush valve is most often

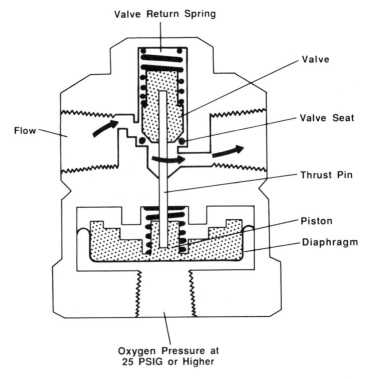

Valve Return Spring

Valve

Valve Seat

Flow

Thrust Pin

Piston

Diaphragm

Oxygen Pressure at
25 PSIG or Higher

FIG. 2. Diagrammatic cross section of an oxygen pressure sensor shutoff valve. If the oxygen supply pressure drops below 50% of normal, this valve stops the flow of all gases except oxygen. (Reprinted with permission of Ohmeda, 1985. The BOC Group, Inc., Madison, WI.)

used when the anesthestist is manually ventilating the patient, and the bag is not inflating as fast as needed (usually due to leakage around the mask). Since this valve shunts only 100% oxygen into the system, one must realize that if used excessively during an inhalation induction, the process may be delayed due to the dilution of anesthestic agent. If the valve malfunctions and remains in the open position, or the operator depresses it for an extended period of time, the possibility exists of overinflating the patient's lungs.

Second Stage Pressure Regulator

This pressure regulator is used in the system to assure that a constant pressure of gas is delivered to the flowmeters (Fig. 1). If this valve were not in place, every time a fluctuation in delivery pressure occurred, the flow through the flowmeters would change. This regulator steps down the pressure from 40 to 60 psi to ~ 16 psi. In the case of nitrous oxide there may or may not be a second stage regulator present. If there is not, then the pressure directed to the flow control valve at the flowmeters is ~ 50 psi.

Flowmeters

The pressure of oxygen at this point is ~ 16 psi and that of nitrous oxide is ~ 50 psi (possibly less if a second stage pressure regulator is present). Each individual glass flowmeter is ground and individually calibrated with its float. For this reason, floats and tubes are not interchangeable. The flowmeters are tapered in the grinding process and the diameter at the upper end is slightly larger than at the lower end (Fig. 3). With this design, the amount of gas flow around the float increases as the float is raised in the flowmeter. The flow control knob is attached to a needle valve. Turning the knob clockwise increases the flow and counterclockwise decreases it. The most recent anesthesia machines are designed to provide, whenever the machines are "ON," a minimum oxygen flow of approximately 300 ml/min, even when the control knob is in the extreme counterclockwise position. This safety feature is designed to provide a flow of oxygen equal to the rate of minimum oxygen consumption. The ANSI machine standard requires that the oxygen flowmeter be on the extreme right of the bank of flowmeters. The flow control knobs are color coded for easy identification; for example, green for oxygen and blue for nitrous oxide. In addition, the oxygen flow control knob has a unique "fluted" shape (see Fig. 3) which is different from the others. This distinctly-shaped knob is designed to help the anesthetist positively identify the oxygen control knob by touch.

The accuracy of flowmeters has been examined by several investigators. The results indicate that flowmeters may be inaccurate at settings between 0 to 14 L/min. Therefore, an oxygen analyzer should always be used to avoid delivering a hypoxic mixture. The flowmeters on Drager's Narkomed 2A are certified to be accurate within ± 3% of full scale, at 20°C and 760 mm Hg barometric pressure. Similar standards of calibration are performed by all manufacturers. Nonetheless, inaccuracies have been found in some flowmeters and therefore, an oxygen analyzer should be used in order to avoid delivering a hypoxic mixture, particularly at low flows.

Recent anesthesia machines feature low and high range oxygen flowmeters which connect in series and are controlled by a single knob (Fig. 4). The low flowmeter is calibrated from 100 to 1,000 ml/min, and the high flowmeter is calibrated from 1 to 12 or 15 L/min. An old design of tandem flowmeters had separate knobs for low and high flow control, but for obvious safety reasons the one-knob design is more desirable.

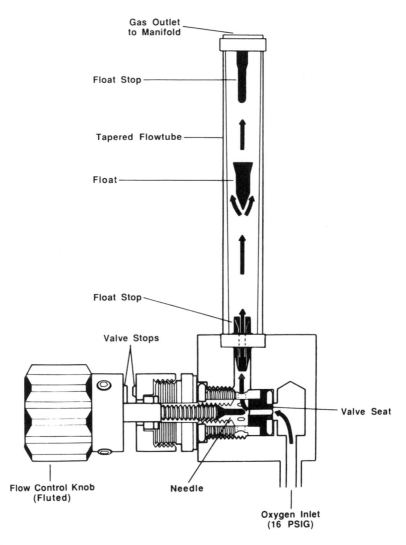

FIG. 3. Diagrammatic cross section of an oxygen flowmeter. Note the tapered shape of the float. (Reprinted with permission of Ohmeda, 1985. The BOC Group, Inc., Madison, WI.)

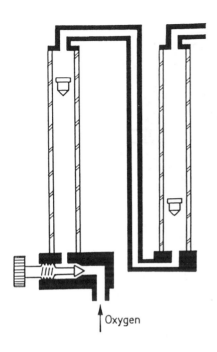

Oxygen

FIG. 4. Diagram of a low and high range oxygen flowmeter in series and controlled by a single knob. (Reproduced with permission from P. Schreiber (1984): *Anesthesia Systems: Safety Guidelines.* North American Drager. Telford, PA.)

Newer machine designs also incorporate devices which alarm or will not allow hypoxic mixtures of oxygen and nitrous oxide.

Vaporizer

Calibrated vaporizer(s) are located downstream from the flowmeters (Fig. 1). After ascending the flowmeters, oxygen and nitrous oxide become thoroughly mixed as they flow through the common gasline approaching the vaporizer. The fresh gas enters the vaporizer through the fresh gas inlet, and soon thereafter a bypass mechanism directs a portion of the stream into the vaporizing chamber where it becomes saturated with anesthetic vapor (Fig. 5). The bypass mechanism is functional over a wide range of flows; typically newer vaporizers demonstrate linear output with flows ranging from .5 to 15 liters. There also exists a temperature compensating device which functions to increase the flow into the vaporizing chamber at low temperatures and to decrease it at higher ones. The fresh-gas that was diverted around the vaporizing chamber mixes with the saturated gas in the mixing chamber and travels out through the fresh-gas outlet.

Technological advances in agent-specific vaporizers have made them reliable, accurate, and easy to use. Vaporizers on newer anesthesia machines are connected in series via a specially designed manifold known

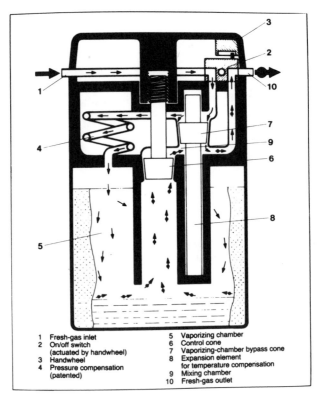

1	Fresh-gas inlet	5	Vaporizing chamber
2	On/off switch	6	Control cone
	(actuated by handwheel)	7	Vaporizing-chamber bypass cone
3	Handwheel	8	Expansion element
4	Pressure compensation		for temperature compensation
	(patented)	9	Mixing chamber
		10	Fresh-gas outlet

FIG. 5. Diagram of a precision vaporizer illustrating the direction of fresh gas, so only a portion of it becomes saturated with anesthetic vapor. The proportioning of the fresh gas flow is determined by the percent of anesthetic selected on the dial on the vaporizer. (Reproduced with permission from *Operating Instructions Vapor 19.n.* 11th ed., 1988 Dragerwerk AG., Luebeck, F.R.G.)

as an exclusion system. This makes it possible to have only one vaporizer on at a time. However, there are many older machines in use today that do not have this exclusion system in place; therefore, the possibility exists of administering more than one volatile anesthetic to the patient.

Factors Affecting Vaporizer Output

The use of free-standing vaporizers brings into consideration several common problems. It is possible in some instances to reverse the fresh-gas connections, thereby reversing the flow of gas through the vaporizer; an arrangement that has been reported to increase the output drastically. This free-standing arrangement also increases the possibility of tipping the vaporizer. When a vaporizer is tipped beyond 45°, the possibility exists of liquid agent spilling into areas other than the vaporizing chamber. With the volatile anesthetic agent in other areas of the vaporizer, the output may become unpredictably altered. Drager recommends that when their vaporizer is tipped beyond the allowable limits, it should be flushed out by running 10 L/min of gas with the concentration dial on the highest setting for a period of up to 20 minutes. The Cyprane Tec 4 vaporizer is designed with a baffling system that allows the vaporizer to be tipped 180°. It is recommended, however, that if a vaporizer has been tipped, its output should be verified by an agent analyzer, or flushed out with high flows, before it is put back in use.

Increased vaporizer output can occur with pressure fluctuations in the patient circuit (i.e., from the ventilator or from the oxygen flush). This phenomenon is referred to as the "pumping effect." The pressure fluctuations are reflected back into the vaporizing chamber of the vaporizer and may cause a significant increase in the anesthetic concentration delivered. This effect, however, has been greatly diminished with the more recent designs of vaporizers and machines. Newer designs incorporate unidirectional check valve(s) and internal modifications in the vaporizer that eliminate the pressure fluctuations from reaching the vaporizing chamber.

Vaporizer Filling Mechanism

To eliminate the possibility of filling a vaporizer with the wrong liquid agent, an agent-specific keyed filling device was developed (Figs. 6A,B). This device is color coded to match the corresponding anesthetic agent, and also has slots which align with the notches on the collar of the agent bottle. This method of filling and emptying is slower than pouring directly from the bottle into the vaporizer filler port. These safety devices have lost their popularity with many anesthetists because, in addition to being slower, they may also have a tendency to leak. It is important to always place the vaporizer concentration dial in the "off" position before filling it or the liquid agent will spurt out when the filling port is opened.

Maintenance and Calibration

Vaporizers should be drained of the liquid agent periodically (e.g., weekly) to rid it of any contaminants that may be present. This drained liquid should be properly labeled and discarded. Halothane contains 0.01 percent thymol which is used to improve the stability of halothane. Thymol tends to accumulate in the vaporizer with time because its vapor pressure is much lower than that of halothane.

High concentration of thymol may effect some of the internal compo-

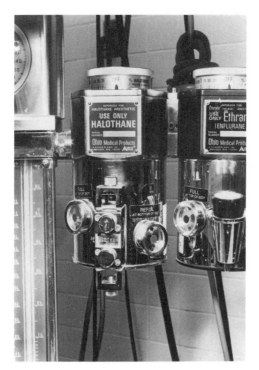

A

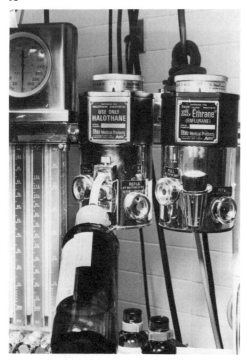

B

FIG. 6. **A.** An example of an agent-specific keyed filling mechanism (halothane) and a nonspecific filling mechanism (Ethrane) on anesthetic vaporizers. Arrows mark the filling ports. **B.** Complete system ready for filling the halothane vaporizer is shown.

nents of the vaporizer thereby altering its accuracy. The increased thymol concentration may be noticed because it gives a brown tint to the liquid in the vaporizer.

PREVENTIVE MAINTENANCE

The purpose of performing routine preventive maintenance on a periodic basis is to prevent possible malfunction or breakdown and to assure optimum performance of the equipment at all times. All anesthesia machine manufacturers offer service contracts which cover preventive maintenance and emergency repairs. Current recommendations are that every anesthesia machine should be serviced every 3 to 4 months. Dr. Clayton Petty, in his book *The Anesthesia Machine,* recommends that this service should be carried out *only* by factory-authorized representatives, and not by hospital biomedical electronic technicians or anesthesia technicians. Having only factory-trained representatives service the anesthesia machines provides additional support for the anesthetist and the hospital as liability would be shared by the manufacturer if an equipment-related anesthetic mishap occurred. Documentation of the service performed on each anesthesia machine, including tests performed and parts used, should be kept on file in the department. In addition to the preventive maintenance records, the department may find it desirable to keep track of modifications and complaints associated with use of the machine. Preventive maintenance must be followed by cleaning and thorough operational checks by anesthesia support personnel and anesthesiologist before each use. The FDA has produced an anesthesia apparatus checkout procedure intended to be performed before delivering anesthesia (Appendix 1). It is expected that this procedure be modified to comply with differences in equipment design and variations in clinical practice. These modifications should be consistent with the procedures and precautions listed in the manufacturer's operators' manual as well as have the acceptance of peer review. Dr. Petty has suggested a short daily anesthesia machine checklist (Table 1) that may be incorporated into the patient's anesthetic record.

TROUBLE-SHOOTING

It is imperative that the anesthesiologist and technician be able to locate and identify problems with the anesthesia machine and patient circuit that may be encountered either during the checkout procedure or during use. Once the problem has been identified, the anesthesiologist or the technician must decide whether they can rectify it or if another machine must replace the malfunctioning one. Because of the liability

TABLE 1. *Pre-use daily check list*[a]

Date _____ Anesthesia Machine Serial # _____

_____ Controls Off	_____ Oxygen Alarm Test
_____ Cylinders Contents Sufficient	_____ Absorber
_____ Oxygen/N_2O Ratio Alarm	_____ Patient Circuit Assembly
_____ Pipeline Supplies	_____ Patient Circuit Leak Test
_____ Gas Flow Controls	_____ Patient Circuit Flow
_____ Vaporizers Filled	_____ Ventilator and Alarm
_____ Machine Leak Test	_____ Scavenging System

[a]Source: Petty C. (1987): *The Anesthesia Machine.* Churchill Livingstone, New York.

concerns, good judgment should be used when attempting to correct malfunctions by anyone other than the authorized factory service representative. Usually the problems encountered deal with tubing, connectors, plugs, etc. that can be easily replaced or adjusted.

Trouble-shooting should proceed in a logical sequence eliminating possible causes until the problem is found. Problems that arise during an anesthetic procedure in the operating room may have to be investigated by someone other than the anesthesiologist administering the anesthetic, thereby allowing the anesthesiologist to direct all attention to the patient. Certainly, any corrective action should be performed under the direction of the anesthesiologist.

Results of a study conducted at an anesthesia meeting indicate considerable room for improvement on the part of anesthesia personnel in their ability to identify anesthesia machine faults. The 179 participants included: 128 anesthesiologists, 22 certified registered nurse anesthetists, and 29 others (dentists, anesthesia technicians, and persons involved in the design, service, and manufacture of anesthesia machines). Each individual was given 10 minutes to identify 5 intentionally-placed faults. The results were as follows: 7.3% found no faults, 3.4% found all faults; the other 89.3% of the participants found an average of 2.2 faults. The professional background did not influence the scores, but those with 10 or more years experience demonstrated increased detection ability. Those problems not rendering the machine inoperable were most often missed.

Appendix 1

Anesthesia System Checkout Procedure

1. Inspect anesthesia machine for:
   machine identification number
   valid inspection sticker
   undamaged flowmeters, vaporizers, gauges, supply hoses
   complete, undamaged breathing system with adequate CO_2
     absorbent
   correct mounting of cylinders in yokes
   presence of cylinder wrench
2. Inspect and turn on:
   electrical equipment requiring warm-up (ECG/pressure monitor, oxygen monitor, etc.)
3. Connect waste gas scavenging system:
   adjust vacuum as required
     if passive, determine free flow to hospital ventilation system
4. Check that:
   flow-control valves are off
   vaporizers are off
   vaporizers are filled (not overfilled)
   filler caps are sealed tightly
   CO_2 absorber by-pass (if any) is off
5. Check oxygen (O_2) cylinder supplies:
   a. Disconnect pipeline supply (if connected), and return cylinder and pipeline pressure gauges to zero with O_2 flush valve
   b. Open O_2 cylinder, check pressure, close cylinder, and observe gauge for evidence of high pressure leak
   c. With the O_2 flush valve, flush to empty piping
   d. Repeat, as in *b* and *c* above, for second O_2 cylinder, if present
   e. Replace any cylinder with less than 600 psig. At least one should be nearly full
   f. Open less full cylinder
6. Turn on master switch (if present)
7. Check nitrous oxide (N_2O) and other gas cylinder supplies:
   Use same procedure as described in 5A and 5B above, but open then close flow-control valve to empty piping
     (Note that N_2O pressure below 745 psig indicates the cylinder is less than ¼ full)
8. Test flowmeters:

    a. Check that float is at bottom of tube with flow-control valves closed (or that min. O_2 flow is so equipped)

    b. Adjust flow of all gases through their full range and check for erratic movements of floats

9. Test ratio protection/warning system (if present:
Attempt to create hypoxic O_2/N_2O mixture, and verify correct change in gas flows and/or alarm

10. Test O_2 pressure failure system:
    a. Set O_2 and other gas flows to mid-range
    b. Close O_2 cylinder and flush to release O_2 pressure
    c. Verify that all flows fall to zero. Open O_2 cylinder
    d. Close all other cylinders and bleed piping pressures
    e. Close O_2 cylinder and bleed piping pressure
    f. Close flow control valves

11. Test central pipeline gas supplies:
    a. Inspect supply hoses (should not be cracked or worn)
    b. Connect supply hoses, verifying correct color coding
    c. Adjust all flows to at least mid-range
    d. Verify that supply pressures hold (45-55 psig)
    e. Shut off flow control valves

12. Add any accessory equipment to the breathing system:
Add PEEP valve, humidifier, etc., if they might be used (if necessary remove after step 18 until needed)

13. Calibrate O_2 monitor:
    a. Calibrate O_2 monitor to read 21% in room air
    b. Test low alarm
    c. Occlude breathing system at patient end; fill and empty system several times with 100% O_2
    d. Check that monitor reading is nearly 100%

14. Sniff inspiratory gas:
There should be no odor or detection of anesthetic agent with agent analyzer

15. Check unidirectional valves:
    a. Inhale and exhale through a surgical mask into the breathing system (each limb individually, if possible)
    b. Verify unidirectional flow in each limb
    c. Reconnect tubing firmly

16. Test for leaks in machine and breathing system:
    a. Close APL (pop-off) valve and occlude system at patient end
    b. Fill system via O_2 flush until bag is just full, but negligible pressure in system. Set O_2 flow to 5 L/min
    c. Slowly decrease O_2 flow until pressure *no longer rises* above approximately 20 cm H_2O. This approximates total leak rate, which should be no greater than a few hundred ml/min (less for closed circuit techniques)

CAUTION: Check valves in some machines make it imperative to measure flow in *c* above when pressure *just stops rising*

17. Exhaust valve and scavenger system:
    a. Open APL valve and observe release of pressure
    b. Occlude breathing system at patient end and verify that negligible positive or negative pressure appears with either zero or 5 L/min flow and exhaust relief valve (if present) opens with flush flow
18. Test ventilator:
    a. If switching valve is present, test function in both bag and ventilator mode
    b. Close APL valve if necessary and occlude system at patient end
    c. Test for leaks and pressure relief by appropriate cycling (exact procedure will vary with type of ventilator)
    d. Attach reservoir bag at mask fitting, fill system, and cycle ventilator. Assure filling/emptying of bag
19. Check for appropriate level of patient suction
20. Check, connect, and calibrate other electronic monitors
21. Check final position of all controls
22. Turn on and set other appropriate alarms for equipment to be used
    (Perform next two steps as soon as practical)
23. Set O_2 monitor alarm limits
24. Set airway pressure and/or volume monitor alarm limits (if adjustable)

Chapter 4

Airway Access and Breathing

ENDOTRACHEAL TUBES

In the sixteenth century, the Swiss alchemist and physician, Paracelsus, attached a fireplace bellow to a tube placed in a patient's mouth to assist in ventilation; and the use of endotracheal tubes had begun. Endotracheal tubes are routinely used in anesthesia and in other areas of medicine where the patient is unable to maintain a patent airway and/or cannot breathe.

The typical endotracheal tube is curved, rounded, and has two ends; the patient end and the machine end (Fig. 1). The patient end is designed to be placed into the mouth and down the trachea, although it may be also passed through the nose and into the trachea. It is beveled to 38 degrees, plus or minus eight degrees of angle, and rounded for ease of insertion according to the American National Standard for Anesthesia Equipment. When viewed with the tube curved up, the bevel is on the left side since most people are right handed. This enables the visualization of the larynx during placement of the tube into the trachea. This is called the Magill Tip. The tip may have a hole near the end called the Murphy Eye, which is designed to evenly direct flow to both lungs and to provide an opening in the event the Magill end becomes blocked. A tube with this type of end is called a Murphy Eye Tube. The end of the tube that protrudes from the mouth or nose is fitted with a part which attaches to a part on the breathing circuit. The tubes usually have a radiopaque line so the position of the tube in the patient can be checked radiographically. If an endotracheal tube has to be shortened, it is done by cutting off the end which protrudes out of the mouth. The tube must have a slippery surface or it must be well-lubricated.

Materials

1. Rubber. The earliest endotracheal tubes were made of rubber. They are still being used, but definitely are being phased out. The earliest

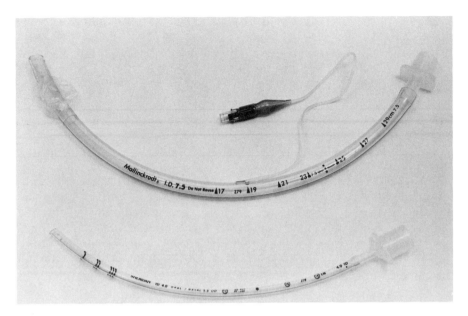

FIG. 1. Cuffed (**upper**) and uncuffed (**lower**) endotracheal tubes. Machine ends are to the right and patient ends are to the left. Note the Murphy Eye on patient end of uncuffed tube.

rubber tubes were rigid, easy to break, and harmful to living tissue. Synthetic rubber reduced these problems, but created new dilemmas as they were too prone to kinking, would break down in the presence of oils and petroleum lubricants, and body secretions would adhere to them.

2. Polyvinyl Chloride (PVC). This is the material most widely used to make modern endotracheal tubes. PVC derived from vinyl chloride varies in substance from manufacturer to manufacturer. The material alone is very hard and brittle, but with the addition of other chemicals can become flexible and nonreactive to other outside agents. Two advantages of modern PVC endotracheal tubes are: they are flexible at body temperatures and mold to the curve of the airway, and they are compatible with body tissue.

3. Silicone. Although silicone is a very expensive material, the silicone tube is gaining popularity. Advantages include: it may be steam sterilized, is a very stable material, throat and nasal tissues do not adhere to the material, silicone is a barrier to body fluids, and is very compatible with any body tissue. Disadvantages include: it is very expensive, is manufactured in limited sizes, and only some have cuffs.

4. Teflon. Teflon is another good plastic material that is compatible with tissue, autoclavable, and slides easily into passages. However, similar

to silicone, teflon is very expensive and has the disadvantage of being very rigid.
5. Nylon. The least used material for endotracheal tubes is nylon. Nylon is a stiff material and can be very toxic to living tissue. However, it is one of the lightest materials used and is very comfortable for the patient.

Cuffed Versus Uncuffed

Some endotracheal tubes have, on the tracheal end, a balloon structure called the cuff (Fig. 1). This cuff can be inflated with air to provide a seal between the tube and the trachea. The inflated cuff prevents the flow of foreign material (e.g., saliva, vomitus) past the tube into the lungs and prevents gas from escaping the tube during positive pressure ventilation. Air is injected into the cuff via a very small tube leading from the machine end of the endotracheal tube to the cuff. A small pilot balloon on the machine end of the small tube indicates whether or not the cuff is inflated. If the pilot balloon is flat the cuff is not inflated, and conversely an inflated pilot balloon indicates an inflated cuff. Cuffs are divided into two categories, a low volume-high pressure balloon and a high volume-low pressure balloon. Low volume-high pressure means a small area of contact and a firmer balloon. This type of cuff is generally used for brief one to three hours intubation cases. The risk of damage to soft tissues increases if this cuff is left in for longer periods of time. The high volume-low pressure cuff has a larger balloon which is softer than low volume cuffs. These cuffs are used for long surgical procedures or for patients who are going to be intubated for days, such as patients admitted to the Surgical Intensive Care Unit or Cardiac Care Unit. The question may arise, "Why are the high volume-low pressure cuffs not used all the time?" The answer is that in short cases the low volume-high pressure cuffs may have a lesser incident of sore throat postoperatively. Also, if the patient is given nitrous oxide, the cuff size may increase two to three times in which case the high volume cuff could expand so much that it could occlude the end of the tube.

There are two indications for use of an uncuffed tube: in people with connective tissue damage from surgery or trauma who would run the risk of more damage to the trachea due to excessive pressure exerted by a cuffed tube, and in small children and infants. Internal diameter of tubes must be reduced to accommodate cuffs. Larger tubes usually are preferred as resistance to air flow is higher with smaller tubes causing increased work in breathing. The subglotic area (the area just below the vocal cords) of children and infants is the smallest part of the airway and is round, whereas the adult and adolescent subglotic area is larger and elliptical. Therefore, in children, an adequate seal can be obtained with a round cuffless tube.

Use of a cuffed tube in children and infants may damage the soft sub-glotic tissue, causing the natural airway to become obstructed on re-moval of the tube. (An uncuffed tube that is too large for the patient may cause the same problem.) Most anesthesiologists use a size of uncuffed tube that just allows a gas leak when the lung inflation pressure is 25 cm water pressure.

Criteria for deciding when to use a cuffed or uncuffed tube is presented in other publications.

Specialty Tubes

Obviously, one tube cannot fit all. Specially designed endotracheal tubes are available to accommodate patients with anomalies and/or cer-tain surgical procedures.

1. Oral/Nasal RAE. The oral RAE (RAE is short for Ring, Adair, and Elwin, the three developers of this tube) is unique in that its shape is bent 90 degrees at the point where the tube exits the patient's mouth (Fig. 2). There are two versions, one used for the nasal passage and the other for oral intubation (Figs. 3A,B). Although designed primar-ily for pediatric use, there are sizes for adults. The oral RAE tube is used when the operational field involves the head area. The tube can be held away and taped to the jaw area allowing the surgeon to main-tain the sterile field and the anesthesiologist to maintain the patient's airway.

   The nasal RAE can be taped to the forehead and also affords the surgeon access to the jaw area, and allows the anesthesiologist use of the nasal passageway without putting unnecessary pressure on the nares.

2. Reinforced or Armored Tubes. This type of endotracheal tube is es-sentially an ordinary tube with a spiral-reinforcing agent, such as wire or nylon, in it (Fig. 2). The importance of these tubes is their resis-tance to bending or kinking. When used in surgery where the head is flexed and manipulated, they prevent compromise of the airway (e.g., neurosurgical procedures involving the head or neck).

3. MLT Tubes. The MLT (microlaryngeal tracheal) tube is specially in-dicated for managing airways in microlaryngotracheal surgery. The tube is offered with internal diameters (IDs) of 4.0, 5.0, and 6.0 mm. The tubes, though small, have the length and cuff diameter of a stan-dard 8.0 mm ID endotracheal tube. The small tube diameter facilitates visualization of the surgical working area and the large cuff provides a firm seal between the tube and trachea. The tube can also be used

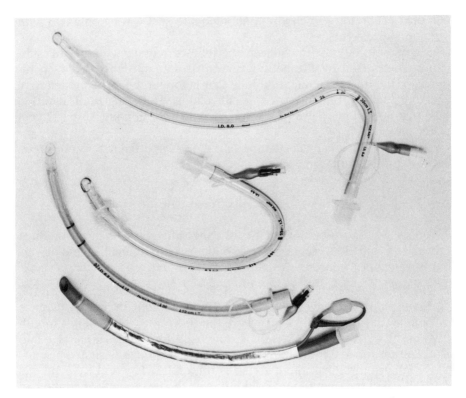

FIG. 2. Four kinds of specialty tubes: nasal RAE; oral RAE; reinforced or armored; and red rubber tube prepped for laser surgery (**top to bottom, respectively**).

in circumstances where the airway has been narrowed by a tumor, or other abnormality, to such extent that the size of endotracheal tube normally used for the patient cannot be inserted. This can be placed orally or nasally depending on the surgical field or the anatomy of the access to the patient's airway.

4. Endotrol Tracheal Tube. The anesthesiologist often has the need to manipulate the end of the tube for proper placement. The Endotrol tube has, attached to the machine end of the tube, a round ring. When moved up and down by a finger, this ring will concurrently move the tip of the tube up and down. This is very helpful in patients with unusual tracheal anatomy (congenital or secondary to trauma).

5. Endobronchial Tubes. Endobronchial tubes are used when it is desirable to ventilate only one of the lungs (Fig. 4). The tubes are designed to be placed directly into the trachea or the left or right mainstem bronchus, and are usually marked accordingly. The tubes are placed into the bronchus and can be checked for position by direct visualization with a fiber optic bronchoscope. The most important use of these

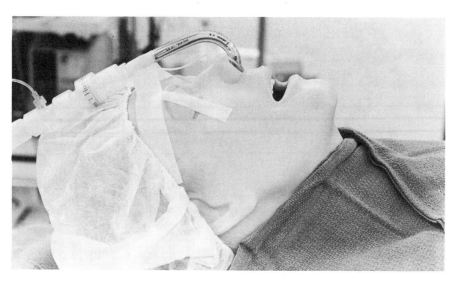

A

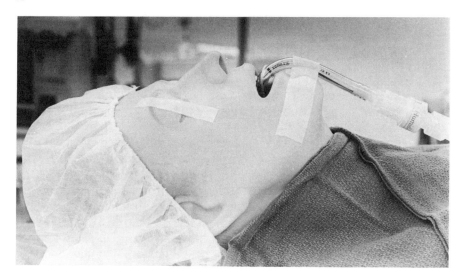

B
FIG. 3. **A.** Nasal RAE in place. **B.** Oral RAE in place.

tubes is for thoracic surgery (e.g., during a lobectomy). The endobronchial tube is placed so the lung section to be removed is not ventilated. The surgeon has a non-moving lung for dissection and at the
same time the anesthesiologist is able to properly ventilate the patient.
Some endobronchial tubes are equipped with a "blocker." The tube
is slid into place and has openings so both lungs can be ventilated

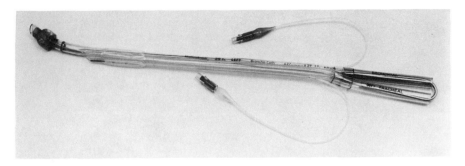

FIG. 4. Endobronchial tube. Note the tube's two lumens. The patient end of the longer portion of this tube is designed to enter the left mainstem bronchus while the shorter portion of the patient end is designed to stay in the trachea.

Then, when indicated, the blocker is moved into position to stop ventilation of the selected lung.

Endotracheal Tube Prep for Use with Laser

Use of lasers to remove or ablate abnormal growths in the head and neck area is expanding. However, the high levels of oxygen normally used during inhalation anesthesia, coupled with the intense heat created by the laser, can cause a potentially hazardous condition. This is the combustion of devices in close proximity to the surgical site, especially the endotracheal tube. "Laser tubes" have recently become available from commercial sources. PVC endotracheal tubes used most often in hospitals are a poor choice for laser surgery. The tubes ignite easily. If they do ignite, they spew out noxious byproducts such as vinyl chloride and hydrochloric acid. Red rubber tubes can withstand multiple laser hits but also can ignite. However, the byproducts on ignition are mineral ash, carbon dioxide, and steam, which are less toxic than the byproducts of PVC ignition; the danger from ignition is primarily due to the release of heat. This tube should be protected by wrapping with metallic tape. The 3M Company manufactures metallic tape one-quarter inch wide which provides suitable protection. It can be purchased through Radio Shack. The thicker metallic tape should be used, not the thinner plastic metallic tape; The latter does not afford the proper protection from a laser hit. The metallic tape actually deflects the laser beam away from the endotracheal tube and thus avoids dangerous ignitions in a patient's throat.

The tube is wrapped, beginning at the cuffed end, and creating a spiral that will not hinder removal of the tube from the tracheal airway (Fig. 2). One must try to wrap slowly and evenly to avoid any kinking of the tape or exposure of any of the underlying red rubber tube. Additional

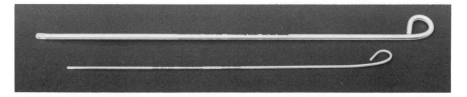

FIG. 5. Two different size stylets used to shape and give rigidity to endotracheal tubes.

precautions should include packing the area with saline-soaked sponges and filling the cuff of the endotracheal tube with normal saline rather than with air. The soaked sponges will absorb laser energy and the saline-filled cuff, if ruptured by the laser, poses no threat and may act as a miniature fire extinguisher.

Stylet

Rigid, plastic coated, metal wires are commercially available, which, when inserted into the endotracheal tube are used to stiffen the tube and hold it in a given shape (Fig. 5). Some anesthesiologists use them during all intubations while others use them only for difficult intubations.

LARYNGOSCOPES

The endotracheal tube usually is introduced through the oropharynx with the aid of a laryngoscope which permits one to visualize the glottic opening and proximal structures. There are two parts to a laryngoscope: the handle and the blade (Fig. 6A). The handle is the part held in the hand; it comes in different sizes. It is circular, and rough so it is easy to grip. Batteries which supply power for the light on the laryngoscope blade are housed in the handle. Most blades form a right angle when attached to the handle; together, these parts are "L" shaped. However, there are some blades that form a "U" when attached to the handle. The connecting part of the blade to the handle is called a hinge (Fig. 6B). A hook-on connector is commonly used so blades can be quickly exchanged. The hinge is fitted with a pin that accepts a slot from the blade. Below the pin is a contact point where electric current flows from the batteries in the handle to the light source in the blade.

The blade is the part inserted into the mouth. Parts of the blade are: base, tongue, flange, web, tip, and socket (Fig. 6C). The base attaches the blade to the handle; it locks in position and makes the electric contact. The tongue is the main shaft of the blade; it serves to move and

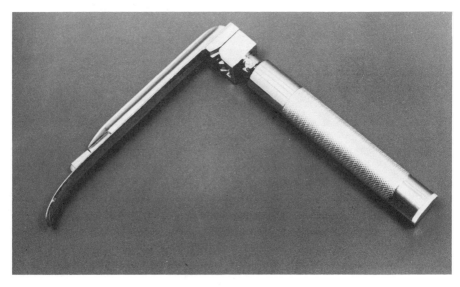

A

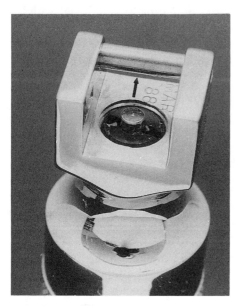

B

FIG. 6. A. Laryngoscope (blade and handle) ready for use. **B.** Close-up of hinge on the laryngoscope handle where the laryngoscope blade connects. Note the pin (**arrow**) running diagonally across the top of the hinge and the contact point below it. **C.** Curved laryngoscope blade. The base that attaches to the handle is on the right. (The blade shown is a relatively new one called the IV MAC. As compared to the standard MAC, the curve of the IV MAC blade is flattened and made concave transversely where the bulb is located. This provides better visualization of the vocal cords. It is available from EpiMed International, 4504 17th Street, Lubbock, TX 79416.) (*Figure continues.*)

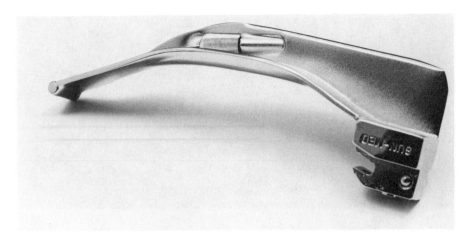

C

FIG. 6. (*Continued*). **C.**

manipulate soft tissues (the patient's tongue), so the larynx can be seen. The flange, attached by the web parallel to the tongue, further guides soft tissue away, thereby providing a "tunnel" for insertion of the endotracheal tube. The tip at the far end of the blade is used to manipulate the epiglottis. The socket holds a light bulb for illuminating the oral cavity.

Blades come in various sizes and shapes (Fig. 7). Blade size is number coded; sizes increases as numeric value increases. Most blades are designed for right-handed people (the handle and blade are held in the left hand and the tube is inserted with the right hand). Left-handed blades can be purchased.

Blade Styles

There are two different types of laryngoscope blades used for intubation: the straight blade and the curved blade. The straight blade is placed under the epiglottis and upward pressure is applied to elevate the epiglottis and expose the glottis. The most commonly used straight blade is called the "Miller." The curved blade is inserted between the epiglottis and the base of the tongue, a forward and upward motion is applied to raise the epiglottis and expose the glottis. The most commonly used curved blade is the "Macintosh." The newly introduced IV Mac is gaining in popularity. The choice of blades is often personal. Advantages of the straight blade include: greater exposure of the glottic opening for better observation of the tube insertion and less need for a stylet. Advantages for the curved blade include: less trauma to the teeth, more

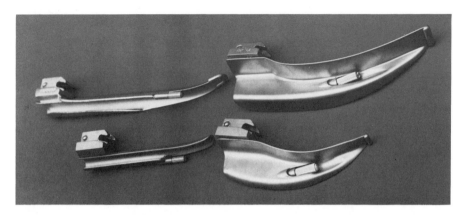

FIG. 7. Two different sizes of laryngoscope blades, straight (**upper**) and curved (**lower**).

room for the passage of the tube, less bruising of the epiglottis and, perhaps, less incidence of coughing and laryngospasms.

Fiberoptic Laryngoscopes

Fiberoptic laryngoscopes with the same general features of the older style blades are available. One difference between the two styles of blades is that the fiberoptic light source is in the handle and not on the blade. Light is delivered to the tip of the blade by fiberoptic bundles. The blades come in the usual sizes in either the curved or straight configuration. The advantages of the fiberoptic laryngoscope are one bulb fits all sizes of blades, the light is of higher quality. Sometimes poor electrical connection causes the light on older styles of blades to flicker; fiberoptic lights do not do this. The biggest disadvantage of the fiberoptic laryngoscope is the cost; it is up to three times that of the old style of blade.

Maintenance and Repair of Regular and Fiberoptic Laryngoscopes

Critical areas that need to be checked regularly include battery charge, functional electrical contact, bulb function, and hinge function.

Most handles use readily available batteries (e.g., size C or AA; there are rechargeable units available). A simple check with a volt meter will determine if batteries are adequately charged. There are two critical electrical contact points, one is the socket area where the bulb is screwed in, the other is the contact point between the blade and the handle. The bulb can become loose and must be tightened periodically; bulbs also may be damaged or just burn out. They can be replaced easily, but care must be taken to use the proper size of replacement bulb. The contact between the handle and the base of the blade can become corroded; remove this corrosion with some fine grain sandpaper. The hinge houses a small pin around which the blade hooks. This can become loose and fall out; an ample supply of pins should be kept on hand. Finally, every day inspection for bent, cracked, and rusted parts of the blade should be made.

Daily maintenance includes proper cleaning of the blades. The blade must be removed and cleaned after each patient use. It should be rinsed in cold water, then scrubbed with a brush with some type of cleaning soap. Two areas are very critical, the tip of the blade and the socket. These areas usually harbor blood and mucous. The blade should be rinsed again in cold water and soaked in 70% ethanol for 20 minutes. Finally, the blade should be rinsed in cold water, inspected, and returned to a bin for reuse. Handles can be used repeatedly unless obviously soiled by body fluids because they usually do not come in contact with patients. If the handle does become soiled, it can be sprayed and cleaned with an antiseptic. Watch for corrosion and oxidation of the electrical contact point.

BRONCHOSCOPES

Intubating Bronchoscopes

Intubating bronchoscopes are designed especially for use by anesthesiologists to perform difficult intubations. Intubating bronchoscopes have an insertion tube; this insertion tube is lubricated and an endotracheal tube is slid over it. The insertion tube is placed into the oral or nasal passage, advanced until the vocal cords can be seen, then advanced further into the airway. Next, the endotracheal tube is slid into place and the insertion tube is removed, leaving the endotracheal tube in proper location. The intubating bronchoscope can also be used to check the placement of the endobronchial tube. Endobronchial tubes are usually placed into the bronchus first, then the insertion tube is inserted to check proper placement.

Physical Description

There are two main types of intubating bronchoscopes, those with the power supply for the light source in the handle of the scope and those with an external power supply. Key parts of the scope include: light source, universal cord, eyepiece, control section, and insertion tube.

The light source provides the illumination for the fiberoptic bundles.

It can be housed directly on the scope itself, with the light bulb and batteries encased in a handle, or it can be a separate box plugged into an AC wall outlet. The universal cord only comes with an external light source. The cord is plugged into an external light source, and optic bundles in the cord transmit the light from the source into the body of the scope. The eyepiece is what the anesthesiologist peers into for visualization of the vocal cords. It usually has an adjustable ring for focussing. The control section, or body, contains three main parts: the control lever, which manipulates the distal tip of the scope up and down; the channel port, which allows air or anesthetic to be introduced; and the suction connector. The insertion tube is the part of the scope which is inserted into the patient. This tube contains three channels, suction, light bundle, and objective lens. The insertion tube has a small diameter and can be slid into endotracheal tubes 4.5 mm and larger. Smaller insertion tubes are available for use in pediatric bronchoscopy.

Cleaning and Maintenance

An intubating bronchoscope must be cleaned immediately after each procedure. Below is the recommended cleaning regime:

1. Wipe insertion tube with gauze.
2. Place distal end in clean water and suction for approximately 10 seconds. Then alternately suction clean water and air several times. Turn off suction device and disconnect suction line.
3. Immerse entire instrument into cleaning solution. Scrub all external surfaces. Remove instrument, place in clean water, and rinse. *Caution:* all scopes are not immersible, check manufacturer's instructions.
4. Insert channel cleaning brush, channel-opening cleaning brush, and suction connector cleaning brush through channels to brush the entire suction line.
5. Connect suction line and alternately suction water and air several times by covering the channel post. Continue to aspirate air for approximately 30 seconds until moisture has been expelled and the channel is dry.
6. Dry all external surfaces of the instrument.

After cleaning, the scope must be disinfected.

1. Immerse fiberscope in disinfectant solution and, using a syringe, pump disinfectant solution through channels. Again, check manufacturer's instructions regarding whether or not to immerse entire scope.
2. Allow instrument to remain in disinfectant solution for recommended period of time, usually 15 to 20 minutes.

3. Suction clean water through the channel until thoroughly rinsed.
4. Thoroughly rinse outside of the fiberscope. Remove the fiberscope from the water and place on a clean, dry surface.
5. Suction air until moisture has been expelled, and the channel is dry.
6. Wipe the outside surface of the instrument dry.

The scope can now be stored for its next use.

Basic maintenance is an exercise in common sense. All parts must be treated carefully; try to avoid all bumps and hits. The insertion tube must not be bent excessively or bumped around. Water soluble lubricants must always be used when sliding on and removing endotracheal tubes from the insertion tube. Avoid direct sunlight, dirt, humidity, and high temperatures.

ANCILLARY EQUIPMENT FOR AIRWAY MANAGEMENT

Magill Forceps

Magill forceps (Fig. 8) are inserted into the mouth and are used to guide the endotracheal tube during nasotracheal intubation.

Oral and Nasal Airways

Different sizes of oral airways and a nasal airway are shown in Figure 9. Nasal and oral airways are used to provide an unobstructed pathway

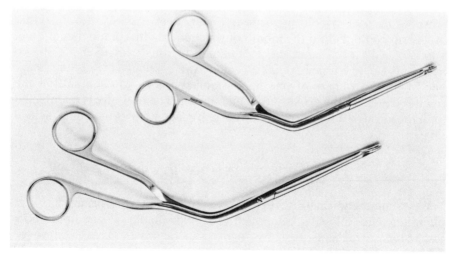

FIG. 8. Magill forceps for adults **(upper)** and for children **(lower)**.

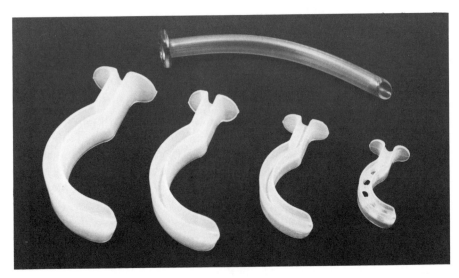

FIG. 9. Nasal airway (**top**) and different sized oral airways.

for air to travel to and from the laryngeal area to outside of the body. Placement is shown in Figures 10A, B, and C. The oral airway also serves as a bite-block, protecting an endotracheal tube from damage that could be inflicted by a patient closing his mouth.

Cricoid Pressure

Application of cricoid pressure is a maneuver used to prevent reflux of gastric contents into the mouth during general anesthetic induction in a patient with a full stomach. Landmarks for this maneuver are shown in Figure 11. The objective is to occlude the esophagus. Pressure is applied with the fingers of one hand simultaneously to each side of the trachea caudal to the cricothyroid membrane. The pressure is maintained until the anesthesiologist confirms correct placement of the endotracheal tube.

EQUIPMENT AT INTUBATION SITES

We recommend that all sites where intubation is performed have, at minimum, the following equipment readily available: selection of endotracheal/nasotracheal tubes; laryngoscope: blades-IV MAC (Improved Vision Macintosh), Miller III, Racz Allen pressure sensitive; BAAM Whistle for confirming blind nasotracheal intubations; McGill forceps;

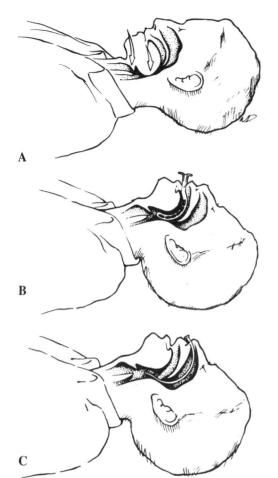

FIG. 10. A. In the unconscious patient, especially in the supine position, soft tissue structures in the back of the mouth will fall back, obstructing the airway. **B,C.** Correctly placed oral or nasal airway, respectively, maintains an open airway. (Reproduced with permission. *Textbook of Advanced Cardiac Life Support.* © American Heart Association, 1987. Dallas, TX.)

stylet, and suction apparatus. Individual preferences, plus any specialized equipment relative to the nature of patient care (e.g., pediatric cases), are supplied in addition to the above.

Note: The Joint Commission of American Hospitals demands that equal patient care be provided at all treatment locations.

BREATHING SYSTEMS

The breathing system is designed to deliver the gases from the fresh-gas outlet of the machine to the patient. There are a variety of breathing systems and a number of ways of classifying them (e.g., Mapleson classification). The most commonly used systems are the circle system, the Bain system and the Jackson-Rees system. For a detailed discussion of

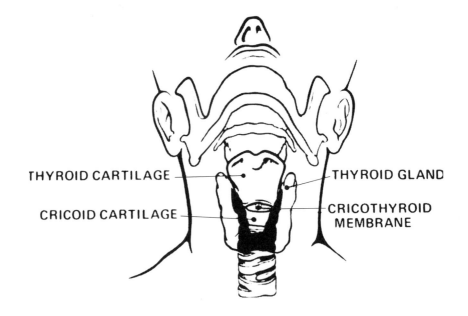

THYROID CARTILAGE

CRICOID CARTILAGE

THYROID GLAND

CRICOTHYROID MEMBRANE

FIG. 11. Anatomical landmarks used to apply cricoid pressure. (Reproduced with permission. *Textbook of Advanced Cardiac Life Support.* © American Heart Association, 1987. Dallas, TX.)

breathing system classification, consult *Macintosh, Mushin, and Epstein: Physics for the Anesthetist* by W. W. Mushin and P. L. Jones.

CIRCLE SYSTEMS

Fresh gas enters the system at the absorber and mixes with the gas that has already passed through the soda-lime canisters. The direction of flow is maintained by the unidirectional valves on the inspiratory and expiratory site. Excess gas is routed through the adjustable pressure limiting (APL) or "pop-off" valve and eliminated through the scavenging system. Commonly present on the absorber is an airway pressure gauge, an O_2 monitor on the inhalation side, and a respiratory monitor on the exhalation side monitor. With this arrangement, the system is defined as either closed or semi-closed, depending on whether the "pop-off" is closed or partially open.

Flow through circuit. Figure 12A illustrates the direction of flow through the system during spontaneous inhalation of the patient. Previously expired gases in the rebreathing bag pass down through the absorber eliminating the CO_2 present, and mix with the fresh-gas from the machine proximal to the inhalation check valve. As the patient begins to

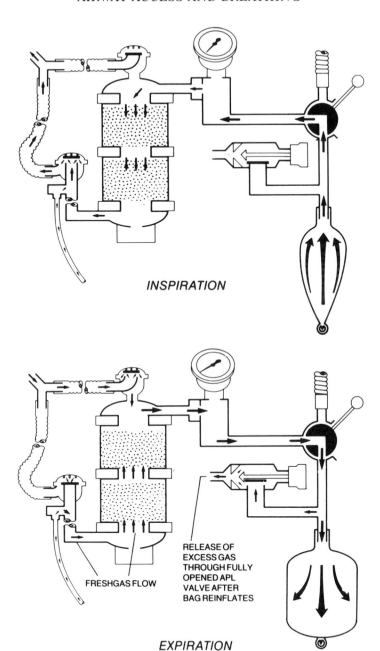

INSPIRATION

A

RELEASE OF
EXCESS GAS
THROUGH FULLY
OPENED APL
FRESH GAS FLOW   VALVE AFTER
BAG REINFLATES

EXPIRATION

B

FIG. 12. Gas flow through a circle system during (**A**) inspiration and during (**B**) expiration. In (**A**) note fresh gas entering system just proximal to the inhalation check valve (**lower left**). (Reproduced with permission from *Operator's Instruction Manual: Absorber Systems,* 1986. North American Drager, Luebeck, F.R.G.)

exhale, the inhalation check valve closes and the exhalation check valve opens allowing the expired gases to enter the rebreathing bag and the excess to be shunted into the scavenging system through the "pop-off" valve (Figs. 12B,13). In controlled mode there are two possibilities; the patient's ventilation can be maintained either by manually squeezing the rebreathing bag or by turning on the ventilator (Figs. 14A,B,C, and D). In the latter case the switch-over valve must be turned as indicated on the machine to replace the rebreathing bag with the ventilator bellows. Some machines also require closing the "pop-off" valve when switching over to the ventilator.

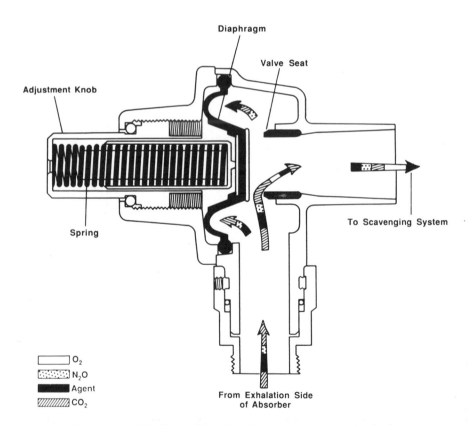

FIG. 13. Diagram of APL ("pop-off") valve. Arrows show route of exit of excess gas from the system during expiration. (Reprinted with permission of Ohmeda, 1985. The BOC Group, Inc., Madison, WI.)

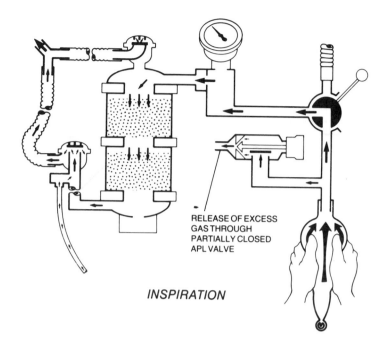

RELEASE OF EXCESS
GAS THROUGH
PARTIALLY CLOSED
APL VALVE

INSPIRATION

A

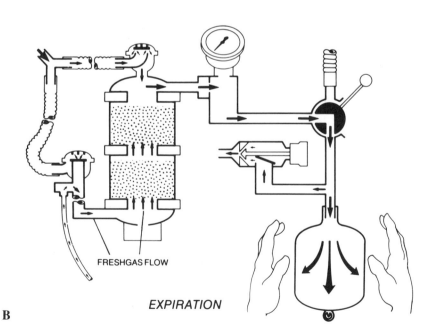

FRESH GAS FLOW

EXPIRATION

B

FIG. 14. Modes for controlled ventilation. (**A**) Manual "bagging" inspiration, (**B**) expiration. (*Figure continues.*)

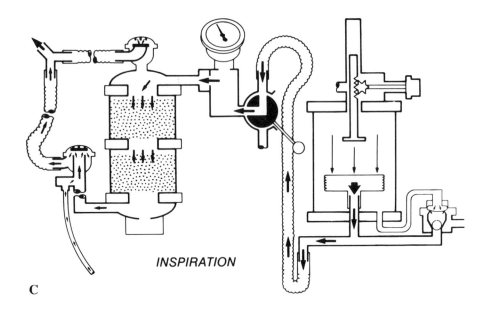

INSPIRATION

C

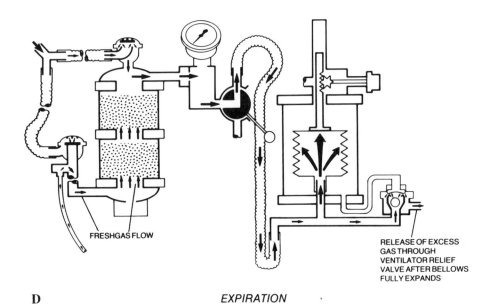

FRESHGAS FLOW

RELEASE OF EXCESS
GAS THROUGH
VENTILATOR RELIEF
VALVE AFTER BELLOWS
FULLY EXPANDS

D   *EXPIRATION*

FIG. 14 (*Continued*).   (**C**) Use of ventilator inspiration, and (**D**) expiration. (Reproduced with permission from *Operator's Instruction Manual: Absorber Systems,* 1986. North American Drager, Luebeck, F.R.G.)

AMBULATORY BAGS

Ambulatory bags, also referred to as ambu bags, resuscitation bags, and bag-mask units, are commonly used in the practice of anesthesia (Fig. 15A). Ambu bags are used to breathe for a patient or to assist a patient's breathing. For anesthesia purposes ambu bags are used during transporting of patients, and in emergencies when there is ventilator failure. An ambu bag is manually operated, self-refilling, and has a one-way valve to control air flow. The common design of an ambu bag includes: an adaptor at one end for connecting the ambu bag to a mask or an endotracheal tube; a patient valve for directing inspiratory and expiratory gases; a self-refilling bag for providing positive pressure ventilation; and a one-way intake valve for allowing gas to enter the bag when it is refilling. An oxygen reservoir can be attached to the intake valve of most bags so oxygen enriched gas mixtures can be delivered (Fig. 15B). The reservoir normally consists of either a reservoir bag that holds the oxygen until it is taken into the ambu bag, or a large open-ended hollow tube that allows oxygen to be held until it is taken into the ambu bag.

Sizes

There are three sizes of ambu bags available: adult, child, and infant. The main difference is the volume of the bag. The volume of bags for adults generally is 1,600 to 2,000 ml; for children generally 500 to 750 ml; and for infants generally 240 to 300 ml. Depending on the manufacturer, the valves may or may not be interchangeable. Sometimes pediatric bags have a special regulator for controlling pressure.

Types

There are a number of different brands of ambu bags that perform well. A wide variety of disposable bags are available for use with infectious cases. Be sure that the ambu bag has a valve that is easy to clean and easy to disassemble, has adequate volume, and is easily handled and compressed. The bag should have a custom-made reservoir that is easily attached.

O_2 Concentrations Delivered

The concentration of oxygen delivered depends on the number of ventilations per minute, the gas mixture delivered, and the flow rate. An oxygen concentration of 21% is delivered if air is used for ventilation;

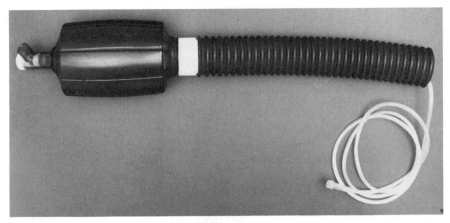

A

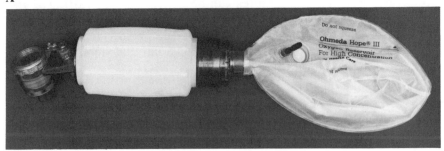

B
FIG. 15. Ambu bag. **A:** Connector for face mask or endotracheal tube, tube for supplying gas, with oxygen reservoir attached. **B:** With oxygen reservoir attached.

when 100% oxygen is delivered to the bag without a reservoir, the oxygen concentration delivered to the patient will be about 40 to 50%. If
100% oxygen is delivered with a reservoir the patient will receive about
100% oxygen.

Applying PEEP

PEEP (positive end-expiratory pressure) is used when it is desirable
to prevent airway pressure reaching 0 during expiration. It is used to
keep alveoli expanded throughout the respiratory cycle. PEEP is used
with very sick patients whose alveoli collapse easily. It is possible to
apply PEEP with some ambu bags by putting a PEEP valve, whether it
is a water column or any other type of PEEP valve, on the part of the
ambu bag where expired gases escape. It is essential that any PEEP devices placed in circle breathing systems be checked carefully: put in
backwards, the patient may die.

Operating an Ambu Bag

An ambu bag is used on patients who are not breathing, or on patients breathing spontaneously but in need of assistance. If the patient is intubated, connect the bag to the endotracheal tube. Otherwise, use the ambu bag with a mask. Great care must be taken when ventilating a patient this way, and proper technique must be utilized.

Cleaning and Storage

To clean the ambu bag, disassemble according to the manufacturer's instructions. Place all parts in water with a cleaning soap and scrub lightly to remove any foreign matter. Rinse with water, then disinfect the parts using either steam sterilization, gas sterilization with ethylene oxide, or chemical sterilization. The simplest way of disinfecting the parts is by chemical disinfection. After washing and rinsing the ambu bag, place it in a container of disinfecting liquid, entirely submerge for at least 20 minutes, then rinse bag completely and allow to dry.

Prior to storing the ambu bag, reassemble and attach the reservoir and oxygen tubing so it is ready for use. The ambu bag unit then can be placed in a large, clear plastic bag and hung in an accessible area.

FACE MASKS

If a patient is given a general anesthetic, ventilation is generally controlled via the face mask before and after extubation. The mask should be comfortable and should create a perfect seal. Masks are held over the patient's face either by hand or by a special head strap. Some masks are transparent, which enables the anesthesiologist to view lip color, secretions, or vomitus (should any be present).

Sizes and Types

Masks come in a number of sizes to fit different patients (Fig. 16). A common adult mask is the anatomical mask from Ohio Medical Products. This mask is flexible and is designed to fit the contours of the face. It also has an air cushion that facilitates a good seal between the mask and face. There are some masks designed specifically for pediatric cases, the most common of which is the RBS (Rendell-Baker-Soucek) also manufactured by Ohio Medical Products. This mask is not flexible and does not have an air cushion; but it fits the face in a way that a seal is obtained and ventilatory dead space is minimized. Most of the masks used in anesthesia will be reusable, but disposable masks are available.

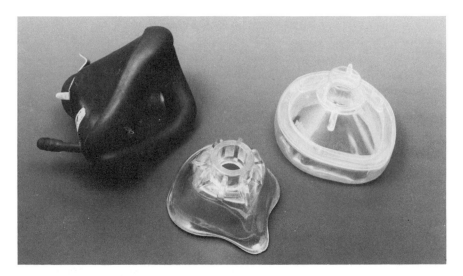

FIG. 16. Three different types of face masks: common adult mask, infant mask, and infant mask with air cushion (**left to right, respectively**).

Cleaning and Storage

Masks come in contact with patient bodily fluids such as mucous and blood. To clean masks, wash in detergent and water. Vigorous scrubbing with a standard scrub brush will remove all foreign material from the mask. As described in the ambu bag section of this chapter, mask disinfection can be accomplished by steam, gas, or chemical sterilization. Masks tend to crack and deteriorate after repeated cleanings so it is important to inspect masks before storage. To store masks, put them in an easily accessible bin according to size.

VENTILATORS

Most patients given a general anesthetic are paralyzed as part of the anesthetic regime, and hence control of ventilation of their lungs is required. This can be done manually by the anesthesiologist rhythmically squeezing and relaxing the reservoir bag on the anesthetic delivery system. Alternatively, the patient can be ventilated mechanically. A variety of ventilators are available. However, the ones most commonly used by anesthesiologists include a ventilator that is part of the anesthetic machine or stand alone devices such as an Air-Shields Ventimeter, a Sechrist Infant ventilator, or a Siemens-Elema 900-C ventilator.

Presently most anesthesia machines come with an attached or built in ventilator. Virtually all of these ventilators are volume controlled. That is, they deliver a present volume regardless of the pressure, ensuring that the patient receives an adequate tidal volume in the presence of changing lung compliance. A pressure cycled ventilator, by contrast, is designed to inflate the lungs to a predetermined pressure and this tidal volume may vary considerably with changing compliance.

How much gas the ventilator delivers with each inspiratory cycle (tidal volume) and the number of respiratory cycles per minute (inspiration, expiration; respiratory rate) are important settings on a ventilator. The inspiratory time: expiratory time ratio can be adjusted on most machines and some allow application of positive and expired pressure (PEEP). Safeguards to prevent over-pressurization of the lungs are provided.

An excellent description of ventilators that are an integral component of the modern anesthetic machine is provided in *The Anesthesia Machine* by Clayton Petty. These ventilators, which are powered by both electrical and pneumatic sources, have two functional parts, a control box and a bellows assembly. Components of the control box integrate the electrical and pneumatic sources that drive the bellows assembly. The bellows assembly can be conceptualized as a bag in a bottle. Anesthesia gases for the patient are contained inside the bellows. During the inspiratory phase, oxygen enters the space between the bellows and the walls of the assembly, forcing gas from the bellows to the patient. Bellows fill during the expiratory phase of the respiratory cycle. Ventilators not integrated into the anesthesia machine used by anesthesiologists work on essentially the same principles just described. Anesthesia gases from an anesthetic machine are routed to the ventilator.

Most recent designs of ventilators used in combination with anesthesia machines have "ascending bellows," which means the bellows rise during the expiratory phase of the respiratory cycle. This design has met with very favorable reviews from anesthesiologists because the ventilator itself is a kind of disconnect alarm. If there is a disconnection anywhere between the ventilator and the non-breathing patient, the bellows will fail to ascend properly during expiration. Individuals who use low-flow or closed circuit anesthesia use the ascending bellows ventilator as a quick guide as to whether or not they are providing enough flow to the patient.

Operation manuals for the various ventilators detail how to direct gas flow through them, how to maintain them, and how to trouble-shoot if they malfunction. All anesthesia ventilators should be included in the anesthesia machine quarterly preventative maintenance contract. Since the inside of the bellows is within the patient breathing circuit, some users feel that the bellows should be cleaned between every case. This probably is not commonly done. It is recommended that, at minimum,

TABLE 1. *Problems with mechanical ventilatory devices reported to the FDA*
between 1976 and 1980 (total number of reports = 280)[a]

Problem	Percent of reports
Problems with breathing circuit	40
Electric circuit failure	14
Mechanical failure	14
Failure of controls, indicators, and alarms	14
Variety of miscellaneous, less frequent problems	18
Total	100

[a]Source: Feeley, P.W. and Bancroft, M.L. Int. Anesthesiol. Clin. 20:83, 1982.

the bellows be air-dried overnight by disconnecting the ventilator hose to the patient circuit at the end of the day.

What problems are generally encountered with ventilators? Problems with mechanical ventilatory devices reported to the FDA between 1976 and 1980 include: problems with breathing circuit, electric circuit failure, mechanical failure, and failure of controls, indicators, and alarms (See Table 1).

Requirements for tidal volume vary considerably from the premature infant to large adults. Since it is difficult to accommodate a wide range of tidal volumes with one machine, machines for infants and children, and for adults are available. The Air-Shields Ventimeter comes with adult and infant bellows. The Sechrist Infant ventilator is commonly used on infants. The Siemens-Elema 900-C ventilator is suitable for infants as well as for adults.

Chapter 5

Vascular Access: Catheters and Guidewires

VASCULAR CATHETERS

There are at least three different approaches to catheterizing blood vessels. One approach is the catheter through the needle method as illustrated in Figure 1. A second approach, illustrated in Figure 2, is the catheter over guidewire technique. Another method is the catheter over the needle illustrated in Figure 3. The catheter over the needle is probably the one most routinely used for intravenous access. The catheter through the needle or over guidewire approach generally is used when inserting catheters that are threaded through the peripheral vascular tree to central blood vessels (e.g., central venous catheters). It would be quite an extensive list of the manufacturers of vascular catheters and guidewires, or all of the catheters and guidewires commercially available. Some of the major brand names and a brief description of how to use certain catheters and guidewires are discussed here.

Sir Christopher Wren is credited with the first successful attempt at cannulation of the venous system. From Wren's time to the present, development of solutions for intravenous (IV) use and of vascular access technology, as well as the evolution of more potent drugs has made the practice of intravenous therapy more sophisticated. The IV route is the fastest method of eliciting a therapeutic response in most cases. It is also the most dangerous.

The purpose of vascular cannulation is to provide an access to the venous or arterial part of the cardiovascular system. Once access has been established, it is possible to provide fluids, drugs, and blood products. It is also a means of obtaining blood for phlebotomy, analysis, or for blood donation. Vessel cannulation is also an excellent tool for measuring central venous pressure from the superior vena cava and arterial pressures (e.g., from the radial artery).

IV catheters range in size anywhere from 24 gauge-¾ inch to 10 gauge-3 inch. The larger the gauge, the smaller the bore and lumen of the cath-

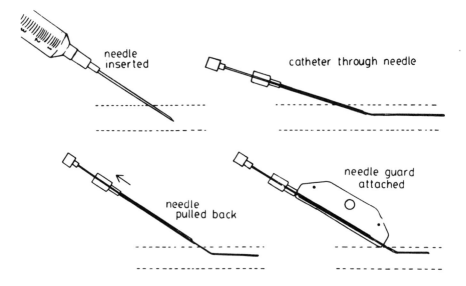

FIG. 1. Through the needle catheter insertion technique.

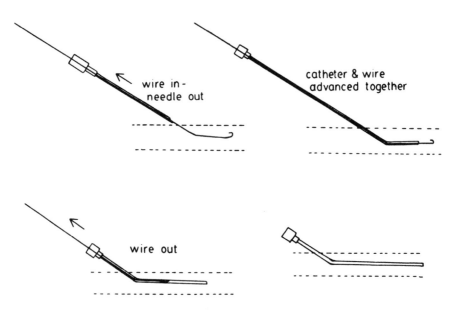

FIG. 2. Catheter over guidewire approach.

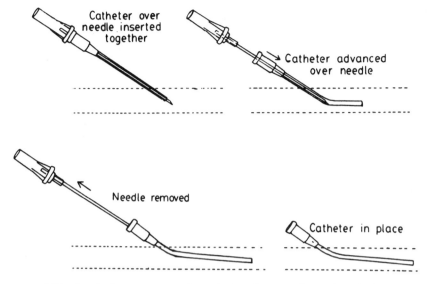

FIG. 3.   Catheter over needle technique for vascular catheterization.

eter. Over the needle catheters have two parts, the insertion needle and the catheter. The insertion needle is made of fine metal and has a bevel tip that is extremely sharp. This makes insertion smooth and easy and does not tear or core the skin.

The catheter fits over the insertion needle and has a tapered body and a hub. The hub is usually color-coded for quick identification of size and gauge. The material content and color code vary from company to company. The majority of the catheters contains a radiopaque covering so it can be seen radiographically. Materials used to manufacture over the needle catheters must be rigid, non-reactive with tissue, non-thrombogenic, and easily sterilized. A particular problem with over the needle catheters is "peel back" (i.e., instead of following the needle through the skin and into the blood vessel, the catheter tip stops at the skin entrance and the catheter compresses onto the needle shaft).

A luer lock fitting is constructed on the end of the catheter so a heparin adapter or other connector can be secured into place. This luer lock looks somewhat like the mouth of a jar without the lid, and is called the female end. The male end can then be twisted on and locked into place. Most, if not all, catheters have a clear chamber on the non-sharpened end to permit visualization of flashback (i.e., the appearance of blood in the hub as soon as the needle enters a blood vessel). (See Fig. 4.)

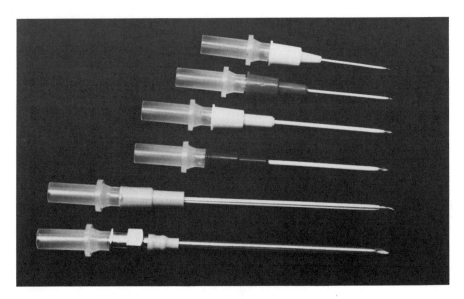

FIG. 4. Examples of various sizes of over the needle catheters: 24, 22, 20, 18, 16, and 14 gauges. (**Top** to **bottom, respectively**). Note clear chamber for opening flashback. Also note all of the catheters have a plastic hub with the exception of the 14 gauge needle, which has a metal one.

Examples of Commercially Available Catheters

Critikon, a division of Johnson and Johnson, makes Jelco and Cathlon IV catheters. Cathlon catheters have a metal hub which is designed to optimize the securing of connections to IV tubing during surgery or long-term catheterization, and grooves for suturing to the skin. Both the Jelco and the Cathlon catheters are made of a transparent virgin teflon. Virgin teflon minimizes drag and patient discomfort, making the insertion smooth. The flashback is immediately evident. The Cathlon catheters come in three configurations: transparent, radiopaque, and striped radiopaque. The striped radiopaque has encapsulated stripes of barium fill for easy x-ray visualization.

Jelco IV catheters have thinwalls. The lumen of thinwall cannulas are larger and flow capabilities are greater as compared to other teflon IV catheters of the same gauge. Hence, smaller gauge catheters can be used if they have thinwalls.

Since the use of a smaller gauge catheter results in less contact with the vessel wall, the risk of mechanical irritation and resulting complications are reduced. The smaller gauge also permits the use of a greater number of vessels, a particularly important factor during long-term IV therapy.

Jelco IV catheters, unlike the Cathlon, come in two configurations: the radiopaque and the striped radiopaque. Transparent Jelco IV catheters are not available; plastic hubs are color-coded to facilitate rapid identification of catheter size. Jelco IV catheters have a high degree of flexibility, and can be bent to considerable extent without distortion of the lumen and subsequent obstruction of fluid flow. The radiopaque cannula contains a high concentration of barium fill for good x-ray visualization.

Jelco IV catheter kits are prepackaged in sterile trays. These kits reduce risk of patient infection from cross-contamination and save the time otherwise required to gather components from a dressing cart or supply room. The kit contains everything needed to perform an IV catheterization: catheter placement unit, tourniquet, providone iodine prep capsule, alcohol swab, $2'' \times 2''$ gauze sponges, Band-Aid brand adhesive bandage, patient identification label, tape, and providone iodine ointment. The kit comes in a sterile, tamper-proof, puncture resistant, peelable-seal package that is color-coded to facilitate rapid identification of catheter gauge. Three other Jelco products are also available on the market:

1. Jelco Intermittent Injection Cap provides a resealable injection site. It is transparent, and has a universal luer lock which ensures secure attachment to the IV catheter. It is an ideal heparin well and a site for repeated injections. The injection site is resealable and can be readily removed to attach conventional IV sets to the catheter.
2. The Jelco IV Stylet maintains a patient IV line and eliminates the cost of re-do procedures. It luer locks in place on both the Jelco and the Cathlon IV catheters. The stylus helps prevent thrombus formation in the catheter lumen and eliminates the need for heparin. It is radiopaque and color-coded for gauge identification. It can be easily removed for intermittent therapy.
3. Jelco 5 Micron Filter Needle is very effective in removal of particulate contaminants. It helps prevent thrombophlebitis, microemboli, and granulomas caused by glass particles or rubber stopper fragments. It has excellent flow rates and a choice of a 19 gauge or 20 gauge needle.

Deseret. Deseret Medical has three basic brands of IV catheters: Angiocath, Novalon, and Insyte. Tips of Angiocath and the Novalon catheters are finely tapered and lubricated to resist deformation. Deseret claims to be the first manufacturer of disposable IV catheters to use color-coded catheter adapters. Both the Angiocath and the Novalon IV catheters have the luer lock adapters for secure connection.

The Novalon catheter has six fully encapsulated radiopaque stripes. No radiopaque particles are exposed on the surface because of the encapsulation of the radiopaque material. The flashback chamber is large and clear for immediate visual confirmation of the primary flashback.

Deseret small bore catheters are less likely to fill the vessel, which helps to assure a more natural flow around the catheter.

The Deseret Insyte IV catheter is made of a unique vialon material, which provides even a greater catheter tip integrity. Vialon material is strong enough to allow thinwall construction, providing superior flow rates with fewer splits, cracks, and peelbacks than thinwall teflon catheters. Vialon remains firm upon insertion, but becomes pliable inside the body, a feature which reduces vessel damage during long indwelling times. Similar in formation to the unique polymers used in artificial organs, arterial grafts, and central line catheters, vialon promotes extended use, and reduces the possibility of irritation and thrombus generation. The insyte catheter is also available with wings for suturing into place.

Terumo. Terumo's Surflo, a recent brand of IV catheter, is constructed of virgin ethylene tetrafluroethylene (ETFE), a fluoroplastic material known for its strength. Both needles and catheters have been processed with medical grade silicone to assure smooth venipuncture.

Abbott. Abbott provides the Venicare System with catheter tips tapering as thinly as possible without sacrificing penetration force, plus virtual elimination of catheter "curl-back" to minimize patient trauma. Two styles of indwelling intravenous catheter are available: Abbocath-T and Clear-Cath.

Also available are the original Butterfly winged infusion sets. These sets make venipuncture easier with automatic alignment of needle in bevel-up position, firm needle control, elimination of needle roll during insertion, and better positioning. After venipuncture, the wings spread flat to provide a firm anchor for taping. Since there is no bulky needle hub to tape down, there is less chance for pressure irritation to develop. Short needle shaft, ultraflexible tubing in regular or short length, and firm anchorage minimize possibility of needle movement within the vein.

Intravenous Catheter Insertion Techniques

1. Wash hands thoroughly and put on sterile gloves, then apply a tourniquet to the extremity and select a vein. To further dilate the vein; 1) have patient clench fist, 2) tap vein lightly with finger, 3) allow arm to hang over side of bed, or 4) apply warm soak to arm for 10 to 20 minutes.
2. Cleanse site with an acceptable antiseptic using a moderate amount of friction. Swab outward in a circular motion. Allow antiseptic to dry thoroughly. Area should not be repalpated.
3. With thumb, anchor the vein below the site of insertion, and pull the skin taut.
4. Hold the flash chamber, not the color-coded hub of the catheter unit. This helps prevent potential insertion problems.

5. With the needle bevel side up over the vein, pointing in the direction of blood flow, use a 15 degree angle for superficial veins and a 25 to 30 degree angle for deeper veins.
6. Insert needle and catheter through the skin and into vein, observing for flashback of blood in flashback chamber. *Caution:* Flashback may occur before catheter tip has also entered the vein. Do not use flashback as a signal to withdraw the needle.
7. Lower the needle until it is almost flush with the skin to avoid puncturing the opposite wall of the vein, and advance the needle and catheter ¼″ further to establish catheter tip in the vein.
8. Stabilize the flash chamber and gradually advance the catheter off the needle until it has entered the vein up to the hub. Release tourniquet.
8a. Alternative Step 8. Advance the catheter slightly to fully sheath the needle tip. The needle serves to reinforce the catheter tip; the catheter tip prevents needle penetration of the vein wall. Holding both hub and flashchamber, thread the needle-supported catheter into the vein up to the hub. Release tourniquet.
9. Place sterile 2″ × 2″ gauze sponge under hub of catheter, withdraw needle from catheter and observe for flow of blood onto gauze to verify proper placement of catheter. *Note:* If catheter does not thread smoothly and/or blood flow ceases, remove catheter and needle together, apply pressure to site, and attempt venipuncture in another site using a new device. Never reinsert the needle into catheter since the needle tip may sever the catheter.
10. Connect administration set which has been previously cleared of air to catheter hub. Open clamp and observe for free flow of fluid before adjusting to proper flow rate. Remove gauze and secure catheter.

There are two popular techniques for securing intravenous catheters: one employing a standard bandage, the other a transparent dressing (Fig. 5).

1. Begin by placing a narrow ¼″ piece of tape under the catheter hub, adhesive side up.
2. Fold one end of the tape diagonally across the hub, being careful not to cover the insertion site or administration set connection, and press firmly to skin.
3. Cross the remaining end of the tape over the first, again avoiding the insertion site and set connection, and press to the skin.
4a. Using an adhesive bandage, cover insertion site and hub, leaving hub end clear to facilitate line connection. A 2″ × 2″ gauze sponge may be taped down in place of an adhesive bandage. Complete procedure by following steps 6 to 8.
4b. If transparent dressing is used, the objective is the same. Cover the insertion site and catheter hub, leaving the hub end clear to facili-

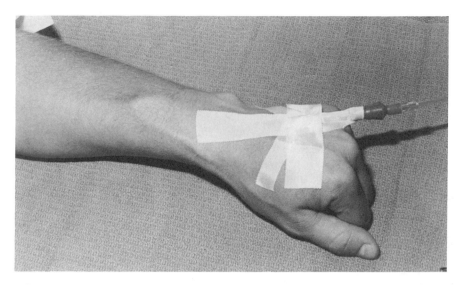

FIG. 5. Illustration of a proper technique for securing an intravenous catheter using a standard bandage.

tate line connection. Semipermeable dressing permits the site to "breathe" and be examined, yet is a barrier to bacteria.
5. Pinch the transparent dressing around the catheter hub to additionally secure the hub.
6. Loop tubing without crimping and tape securely with 1″ tape.
7. Add a length of 1″ tape to further secure looped line. The purpose of the loop is to absorb any pulling on the IV line, thereby preventing catheter dislodgment.
8. Label insertion site, noting the catheter gauge, date and time of insertion, and initials of the person performing the venipuncture. *Note:* Tape should never completely encircle arm, doing so could restrict blood circulation.

Always use aseptic technique (sterile technique) during catheter insertion, care of the insertion site, and manipulation of any equipment used in the administration of intravenous therapy. Inspect all fluid containers before use for signs of contamination (e.g., turbidity).

GUIDEWIRES

Guidewires or J wires come in different sizes. Two basic sizes are 30 French diameter and 30 inch length, or 30 French diameter and 90 inch length. They are a spring wire, with one end shaped like the letter "J", which can be inserted through the needle when placing a catheter such

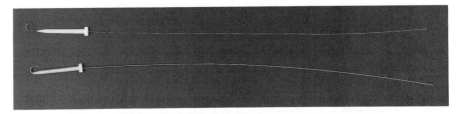

FIG. 6. Two J wires with plastic sheath.

as a central venous catheter or triple lumen catheter. The "J" part of the wire is an extremely soft and flexible spring that will not pierce the lumen of a vein. There is a plastic sheath supplied with the wire that straightens the "J" tip for insertion through a needle and into a vein (Fig. 6). Once this has been done, the plastic sheath is retracted and the "J" is threaded through the vein. After the spring wire is placed through the needle and threaded into the vein, the "J" tip is placed a little beyond where the tip of the catheter will rest. The catheter then can be placed over the "J" wire and threaded into place. Once this has been done, the "J" wire is retracted with the catheter in place.

Radial Arterial Lines

A radial arterial line (ART line) is commonly used when invasive measurement of arterial pressure is necessary. Usually a 20 gauge IV catheter is inserted into the radial artery and noncompliant high pressure tubing is connected to the catheter. A special monitoring transducer cable is set up and connected to the IV. A plug on the opposite end of the cable is connected to the monitor and the transducer is calibrated.

A radial artery catheter kit is available from Arrow International. The kit includes a 20 gauge catheter. Different catheter sizes and configurations are available with a guidewire and introducer needle (Fig. 7). The area is prepped and the introducer needle is inserted into the radial artery. When flashback occurs the guidewire is introduced into the radial artery. After the guidewire is in place, the catheter is slipped off the introducer needle and over the guidewire, and secured in place. The guidewire is then retracted.

Central Venous Pressure Kits

There are many different brands of Central Venous Pressure (CVP) kits on the market today (e.g., Pharmaseal, Burron, Arrow, Kendall, and many more). CVP kits work somewhat in the same way the arterial line

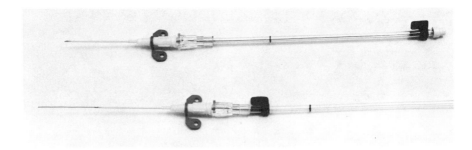

FIG. 7. Arterial catheter, introducer needle, and guidewire. Guidewire still in needle shaft **(top)** and extended maximally **(bottom)**. Ring on plastic shaft marks location of device used to slide guidewire into vessel when tip of guidewire is about to exit the needle tip. Note wings with holes on catheter hub through which suture material can be passed to attach the catheter to the patient.

kits work. Central venous pressures are recorded from the superior vena cava.

The following are the contents and directions for the use of a central venous catheter tray:

one 25 GA × 1″ (2.54 cm) skin wheal needle
one 22 GA × 1½″ (3.81 cm) vessel locating needle
one 18 GA × 2½″ (6.35 cm) TW needle
one 16 GA × 2½″ (6.35 cm) heavy wall teflon radiopaque
catheter over 200 GA introducer needle
two 5 cc syringes
one .035″ (.89 mm) dia × 17¾″ (45 cm) dual purpose spring wire guide
(straight soft tip on one end/"J" tip on the other)
one disposable scalpel (#11 blade)
one straight silk suture
one ampule lidocaine HCL 1%
three 2″ × 2″ gauze pads
four 4″ × 4″ gauze pads
one 16 GA × 8″ polyurethane radiopaque indwelling catheter
one fenestrated drape
three providone-iodine swabsticks
one CSR wrap
one providone-iodine ointment
one vessel dilator

The above is a basic kit. Many different kits are available, and configuration of contents may vary. Most hospitals specify what they want in their kits.

Suggested Procedure for Insertion of CVP Lines

1. Peel open package and remove prep swabsticks.

2. Prep skin in area of anticipated venipuncture.
3. Remove CSR wrapped tray and open to create sterile field and expose kit components for use.
4. Place drape over prepped puncture site.
5. Use 21 GA needle and 5 cc syringe to locate and enter central vein.
6. Attach 5 cc syringe to 16 GA × 2½″ (6.35 cm) catheter introducer. Insert into vein along side of 21 GA locater needle. Remove 21 GA needle.
7. Remove introducer needle. If no free flow of venous blood is observed, attach syringe to catheter and aspirate until good venous blood flow is established. *Caution:* Do not reinsert needle into catheter.
8. Insert desired tip of spring wire guide through 16 GA × 2½″ (6.35 cm) catheter into vein. If "J" tip is used, prepare for insertion by sliding plastic tube over "J" to straighten it. Advance spring wire guide to required depth. *Note:* Advancement of the "J" tip may require a gentle rotating motion. *Caution:* Maintain firm grip on wire at all times.
9. Hold spring wire in place and remove introducer catheter.
10. Enlarge cutaneous puncture site with scalpel. Do not cut wire guide. Use vessel dilator to enlarge site as required.
11. Thread top of indwelling catheter over spring wire guide. (Be certain that sufficient wire guide length remains exposed at the hub end of catheter to maintain a firm grip on wire guide.) Grasp catheter near skin and advance into vein with slight twisting motion.
12. Advance catheter to required position.
13. Hold catheter at depth desired and remove spring wire guide. Attach syringe and aspirate until free flow of venous blood is observed.
14. Connect catheter to intravenous line or manometer.
15. Use suture to secure catheter and/or purse-string insertion site if necessary. Providone-iodine ointment can be used to cover puncture site. *Note:* An 18 GA × 2½″ (6.35 cm) TW needle may be used instead of the 21 GA to locate the vein. The 18 GA needle will pass .035″ (.89 mm) diameter spring wire guide if desired.

Chapter 6

Circulatory Monitoring

ELECTROCARDIOGRAPHY (ECG)

Blood performs an essential role in maintaining the body's vitality and it is important for anesthesiologists to know that the blood pump (i.e., heart) is working effectively. The ECG reveals considerable information about how the heart is functioning; therefore, the ECG is routinely monitored during anesthesia.

The ECG can be readily produced by placing two electrodes directly on the beating heart, but this is rarely practical. Fortunately the ECG signal is radiated outward from its source, the heart. Willem Einthoven identified and standardized the placement of electrodes on the body in a three-point array known as the Einthoven Triangle (Fig. 1). The voltage between two of the three points was originally measured, using the third point as a reference. Later investigators extended the number of measurement arrangements using the right leg as reference. There are now twelve distinct electrode arrays, (ambiguously called "leads") in a complete diagnostic ECG, based on the placement of eleven electrodes (Fig. 2). In any of these leads, the monitor detects the voltage waveform across only two points (or two combined points) at a time. Lead I, II, or III is usually monitored during surgery, although most monitors are capable of recording any of the 12 leads. When the physician needs to analyze variants in the ECG, one of the chest leads (V1-V6) may be preferred, in which case a "modified V5" lead is sometimes used. For this, the electrodes normally used as lead I are positioned on the chest and back in order to emphasize the P- and T-waves (Fig. 3). Another option is to use an esophageal probe as an active electrode, taking advantage of its proximity to the heart (Fig. 4). The principal features of the waveform, recorded via lead II, include: 1) the P-wave which is created as atria cells depolarize, 2) the QRS complex generated by depolarization of ventricular cells, and 3) the T-wave generated by repolarization of ventricular cells (Fig. 5). Deviations from the "normal" pattern (or from the patient's known waveform) may be significant in the course of a surgery, although during general anesthesia over 50% of patients display

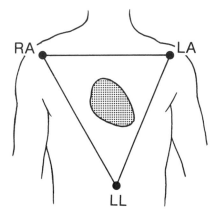

FIG. 1. Einthoven Triangle formed by standardized placement of electrodes on the body in a three-point array. RA and LA = right and left arm respectively. LL = left leg. (Reprinted with permission from P. Strong (1971): *Biophysical Measurements*, 1st edition. Tektronix Corp., Beaverton, Oregon.)

some form of dysrhythmia according to some sources. It falls to the judgment of the physician whether abnormalities in ECG (or any other parameter) represent a significant change in the patient's status that requires action.

The problem of interfacing the ECG monitor with the patient has been the focus of much attention. Electrically, the skin represents a complex opposition to ECG signals. The earliest techniques used saline-soaked bandages to which metal plates were attached, or simple immersion of three limbs in saline-filled metal buckets connected to the measuring device! Later, metal plates coated with electrically conductive paste were used; and eventually the skin barrier was broken by using small needles. While this provided a better signal, needles were painful and involved risks of bleeding and infection. However, sterile needle electrodes are necessary for burn patients if the burn area is where the electrodes are to be placed.

The increased acceptance of ECG monitoring predictably generated a market for disposable electrodes that were electrically competent, non-invasive, and reliable (Fig. 6). One company produces a "back-pad" electrode which incorporates all five electrodes in one foam layer to be applied for monitoring in the OR. This is especially useful for infants and small children. A standard exists which specifies electrical and physical criteria for ECG recording, including acceptable impedance levels (i.e., opposition to varying electrical signals) and "dc offset" (i.e., the voltage created by the gel-to-metal-to-patient interface). Most electrodes depend on a silver-coated metal connector with a gel containing silver chloride to conduct the signal. A metal snap-button on the electrode usually is where monitor cables are attached. The variable in most products is the adhesive and backing material; paper, foam, and cloth are used.

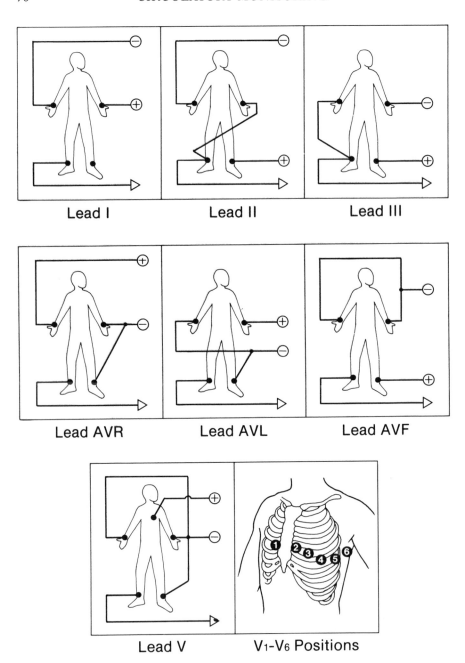

FIG. 2. Standard connections for each of the 13 ECG leads. "+" and "−" refer to the polarity of the active leads, referenced to the "ground" leads. (Reprinted with permission from J. Carr and J. Brown (1981): *Introduction to Biomedical Equipment Technology,* 1st ed. John Wiley & Sons, Inc., New York.)

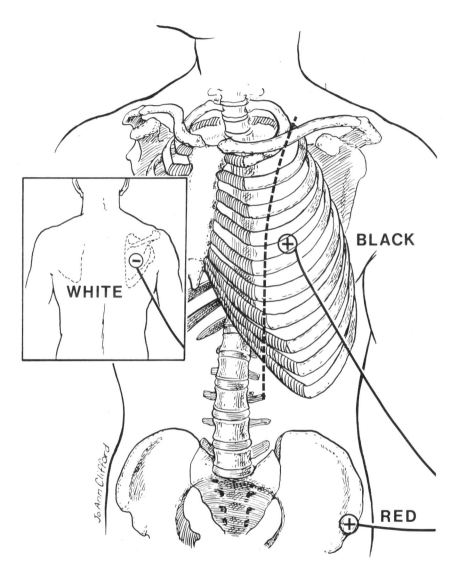

FIG. 3. The "Modified V-5" lead often used in anesthesia. By selecting Lead I at the monitor, the status of the posterior aspect of the heart can be emphasized; selecting Lead II emphasizes the anterior aspect of the heart.

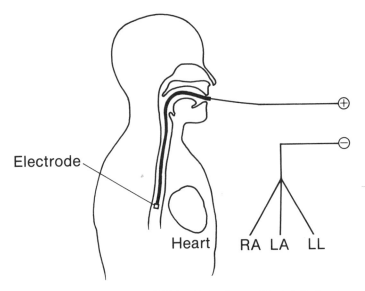

FIG. 4. Diagram of the esophageal ECG lead. As shown, RA, LA, LL leads are joined and connected to the − pole of the recording system and the esophageal lead is connected to the + pole. (Reprinted with permission from P. Strong (1971): *Biophysical Measurements,* 1st edition. Tektronix Corp., Beaverton, Oregon.)

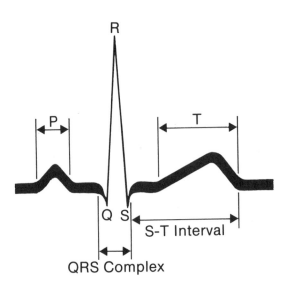

FIG. 5. Idealized ECG waveform showing components recorded during one cardiac cycle. (Reprinted with permission from J. Carr and J. Brown, (1981): *Introduction to Biomedical Equipment Technology,* 1st ed. John Wiley & Sons, Inc., New York.)

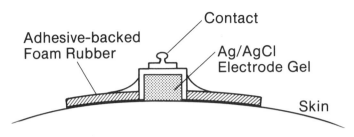

FIG. 6. Schematic of disposable ECG electrode.

The American Heart Association set a standard in the 1950s for the color-coding of the connectors at the five electrode points: right arm, white; left arm, black; right leg, green; left leg, red; and chest, brown. These are used on all monitor connectors and their lead wires.

ECG monitors have evolved from cumbersome vacuum-tube units in the 1950s to the current generation of microprocessor-based multi-function models (Fig. 7). Despite all variations in form and function of monitors that are available, the essential features in any unit are an adequate display of the ECG waveform and adjustable alarms. Almost without exception, the waveform is displayed on a cathode-ray tube (CRT); the standard speed of the trace is 25 mm/sec with most models offering options of half or twice this speed (12.5 mm/sec provides more time span on the screen, while 50 mm/sec provides more detail of the waveform). Most units provide a "freeze" function whereby the ECG can be stopped for further analysis or recording; usually it is relocated elsewhere on the screen while the real-time signal continues. Roughly half of the monitors available incorporate a strip-chart recorder or provide space for an optional recorder. The ability to obtain a "hard copy" of an unusual ECG episode is very useful for clinical teaching purposes and occasionally for medico-legal documentation.

Alarms that can be set by the user are almost universally provided with both an upper and lower heart rate limit. Some models enable the alarms to be defeated entirely, while others cannot be turned off but the volume of the alarm can be decreased. In either case, the alarm status is annotated on the CRT screen in the more contemporary units, often with the heart rate and lead selection. The alarm circuitry of many models automatically triggers the recorder to produce a 15 to 30 second record, which is often annotated with time, date, and lead selection.

The majority of difficulties encountered with ECG monitors originate at the electrodes. The skin must be reasonably clean, dry, and clear of body hair in order to assure good electrode contact. Taking the additional 15 seconds to wipe the skin with alcohol and dry it, or shaving hair if necessary, can save a great deal of time and stress later. Otherwise, ECG

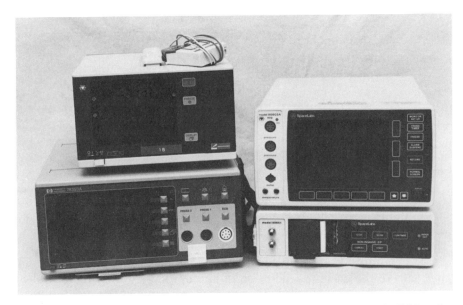

FIG. 7. Representative monitors for ECG plus other function. **Top left:** ECG only, using telemetry (transmitter on top). **Bottom left:** ECG plus two pressure channels. **Right:** ECG, two pressure channels, temperature, noninvasive blood pressure, and recorder.

quality may deteriorate and surgical drapes may prevent access to the electrodes. Some manufacturers provide an abrasive pad on their electrode with which to abrade the skin and assure good signal transfer. Occasionally an electrode will be found whose conductive gel has dried; always ascertain that the gel is wet before attaching the electrode (Fig. 8).

Connecting wires attach to the button on the electrodes via spring-loaded clips; inspect these routinely for damage or wear (Fig. 9). Electrodes and connected wires are often generously dripped or coated with surgical skin prep solutions by nursing staff; this can compromise the adhesion of the electrode. Electrodes can be protected against this risk with supplemental adhesive tape (Fig. 10).

The three most common interferences with ECG recordings are high-frequency signals from nearby electrocautery, 60-cycle (60 Hz); interference from line-operated devices in contact with the patient; and a "wandering baseline" (Fig. 11). Most recent monitors have circuitry which senses and filters out the cautery signal. Modern cautery units are "cleaner" than in decades past, so cautery interference is not the major problem it used to be. Leakage of 60 Hz alternating current from the power line may occur when many devices are in use or if one device has excessive leakage to "ground." Besides compromising the ECG, 60 Hz

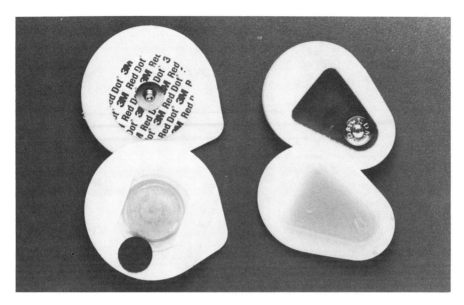

FIG. 8. Standard disposable ECG electrodes. Note small abrasive patch on pad (**left**) used to prepare skin surface before electrode application.

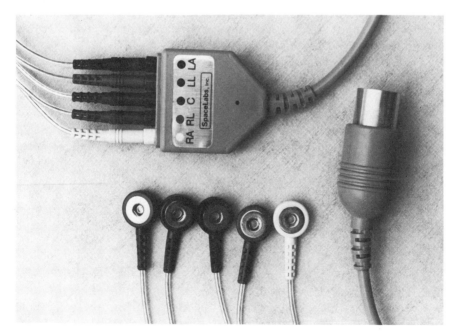

FIG. 9. Typical ECG connector cable and leads. Connector block usually includes a resistor in each lead for electrical safety.

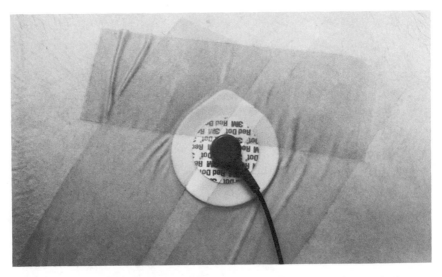

FIG. 10. ECG electrode secured with tape for additional protection against prep solutions or heavy fluid exposure.

interference may imply a threat to patient safety, and should be investigated. Separately unplugging each device in the vicinity will often reveal the source of the problem. Wandering baseline, less threatening but nevertheless annoying, is usually due to a loose electrode, and often occurs in phase with the patient's respiratory movements.

BLOOD PRESSURE MEASUREMENT

Contemporary anesthesia practice allows clinicians to monitor as many as eight or ten different physiologic variables in the course of a typical general anesthetic. Given the choice of monitoring only one of these, many practitioners would readily opt for blood pressure monitoring, however, this is not consistent with the ASA monitoring standards.

In concept, the vascular system might be considered to be a closed plumbing system consisting of two pumps forcing fluid through two networks of vessels (Fig. 12). The pumps are, of course, the left and right heart chambers. The left heart ventricle delivers blood to virtually the entire body through vessels (arteries and arterioles) of decreasing size, after which it returns to the right heart chambers via the venous system. The right ventricle delivers the blood to the lungs from which it returns to the left heart chamber to complete the loop. Unless otherwise specified, blood pressure measurement takes place on the arterial side of this loop. Two further points need be made regarding this plumbing analogy: the pumps perform their work in strokes, so their output is pulsatile; and

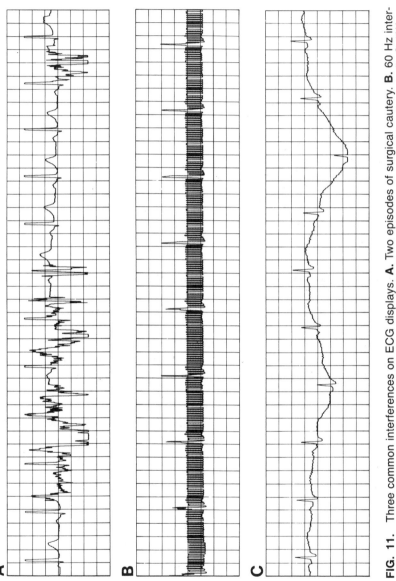

FIG. 11. Three common interferences on ECG displays. **A.** Two episodes of surgical cautery. **B.** 60 Hz interference from adjacent equipment (note that the essential P-, R-, and T-waves can still be discerned). **C.** "Wandering baseline," typical of a loose electrode. Waveform wanders periodically with the patient's ventilatory cycle.

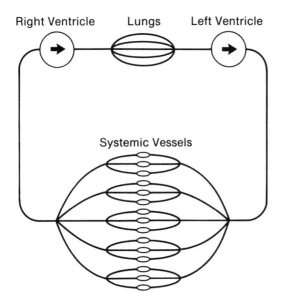

FIG. 12. Generalized diagram of the cardiovascular system.

the plumbing is not rigid but elastic, consisting in part of smooth muscle which can constrict and relax under the body's automatic control.

With this in mind, one can better understand the differing blood pressure waveforms seen at various points in the arterial system. Detected in the largest arteries, the waveform reflects the individual pulses of the left ventricle, and returns almost to zero between pulses. Further downstream, the resistance offered by narrowing vessels results in a constant "back pressure" on which the pulses ride. The peak value of each pulse is the systolic pressure, and the resting pressure between pulses is the diastolic pressure. Mean arterial pressure (MAP) often is used as a generalization of blood pressure status; true MAP is the time-weighted average of the pressure at several points in the waveform. A commonly used approximation of MAP is diastolic pressure plus one-third of the pulse pressure (i.e., systolic pressure − diastolic pressure). The specific shape of the waveform depends upon a number of interacting variables: the stroke pattern of the heart, the size of the vessel, the muscle tone of vessel, and the distance from the heart. One predictable waveform feature is a relatively small second peak occurring on the descending side. This "dicrotic wave", which creates a "dicrotic notch", is held to result from the reflection of some wave energy from the many elastic vessels and tissue downstream.

Blood pressure is almost universally measured in millimeters of mercury column height (mmHg), although the international standard for pressure is the Pascal (Pa). The relative size of one kiloPascal (kPa) (one kPa = 7.5 mmHg) makes it cumbersome for the typical range of blood pressure values. Occasionally "torr" is used in place of mmHg and is 1/760th of the ambient atmospheric pressure and is identical to mmHg if sea level pressure is assumed.

Invasive Blood Pressure Monitoring

Invasive blood pressure monitoring requires the placement of a catheter into a peripheral artery and connection of the catheter to a device that directly measures pressure in the arterial system. This procedure was first performed more than 250 years ago by Stephen Hales who cannulated an artery in the neck of a horse and observed the column of blood that rose above the heart. Direct blood pressure monitoring became widespread among clinicians during the last 15 to 20 years with the advent of open heart surgery. Also during this time, great advancement was achieved in the field of electronic monitoring of the cardiovascular system. Continual improvement in over the needle catheters and improved techniques for inserting and maintaining arterial catheters lowered the incidence of complications with direct blood pressure monitoring, but as with any invasive procedure, there are always associated risks. This chapter will examine and describe the major aspects of invasive blood pressure monitoring, with emphasis on the practical aspects. The reader is urged to consult the reading list at the back of this book to obtain a more in-depth understanding of the technical and theoretical aspects of this procedure.

Currently in the field of anesthesiology, the practice of direct blood pressure monitoring is a very common occurrence; it is an easy way to monitor blood pressure on a beat-to-beat basis. This type of vigilant monitoring is indicated in a variety of patients: for those having open-heart surgery; for trauma or surgical patients in whom a large blood loss is anticipated; for patients with an unstable cardiovascular system; for situations where access to arterial blood is required for blood gas analysis, etc. Many clinicians feel that direct pressure monitoring is the "gold standard" to which other methods of blood pressure determination should be compared. One must remember that pressure does not mean flow; in fact, very high blood pressure most likely represents a decreased flow condition. Return of flow methods for determining blood pressure use an occluding cuff which is inflated to a pressure higher than the systolic pressure, and then slowly deflated. Determination of systolic and diastolic pressure is interpreted through determination of turbulent flow of blood under the cuff. Often the results obtained by this method do not agree with the results obtained by direct intraarterial methods of determining blood pressure. Some studies have shown direct measurements to be higher than indirect measurements, and others show the opposite. Both direct and indirect methods of blood pressure determination have their limitations. Frustrations are avoided not by trying to correlate one with the other, but instead understanding each and the theory behind it.

The transducer and coupling system. The intraarterial pressure monitoring system consists of a catheter placed in the lumen of an artery with the tip directed toward the heart. A coupling system, composed of high pressure tubing and a stopcock for blood sampling, connects the catheter to a pressure transducer. The system also contains a constant infusion device that is designed to infuse normal saline containing heparin at a concentration of two units/ml through the coupling system and catheter to prevent clotting at the catheter tip. The rate of infusion is approximately 3 ml/min when the bag containing the heparinized saline is pressurized to 300 mmHg. The arterial pressure wave is transmitted through the liquid-filled catheter and coupling system to the pressure transducer. This converts the pressure wave into an electrical signal that is amplified, modified, and displayed on a physiologic monitor (Fig. 13). Most monitors display both the waveform and the numeric values of the blood pressure. Systolic, diastolic, and mean pressures are determined in the fol-

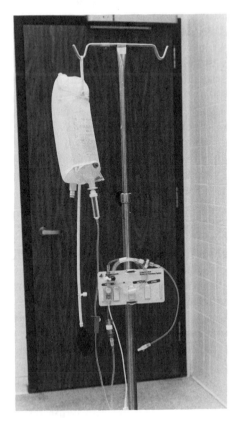

FIG. 13. Intraarterial pressure monitoring system. Fluid-filled plastic bag is pressurized to 300 mmHg by inflating jacket over it with air (via bulb hanging down). Fluid exits the bag and passes through the tubing at approximately 3 ml/min.

lowing manner: systolic is taken as the highest pressure; diastolic as the lowest pressure; and mean pressure is determined by integrating the area under the pulse-pressure wave.

There are a vast number of different types and sizes of pressure transducers, but in recent years disposable transducers have become very popular with clinicians and hospital staff due to their dependability, ease of use, and low cost. Whether using disposable transducers or reusable ones with disposable domes, strict attention and adherence to the manufacturer's recommendations for set-up and calibration should be made in order to avoid inaccuracies caused by bubbles or poor connections.

A few important aspects pertaining to the physical characteristics (i.e., oscillation, damping, resonance or ringing) of the transducer and coupling system should be understood to ensure good results in a given application. Arterial blood pressure oscillates between systolic and diastolic pressure. If the system used to record an oscillating signal is not exactly accurate for recording such a signal, ringing or damping may occur. Resonance is the tendency of an oscillation to increase in amplitude and frequency until a maximum is reached; whereas damping is the opposite. To avoid resonance and overshoot (i.e., "ringing") the transducer and recording system should have a flat frequency response (the ability to respond to pressure changes) of approximately one and one half times the frequency of the waveform to be measured. Arterial pressure waveforms have frequency components that may be as high as 30 Hz; therefore the monitoring system should have a flat frequency response of 45 Hz. Most pressure transducers currently on the market demonstrate a flat frequency response of at least 50 to 100 Hz; therefore the drop in frequency response must come from the catheter and coupling system. As the natural frequency of the pressure monitoring system moves closer to that of the pulse pressure wave, ringing may occur causing alteration of the pressure waveform and overshoot of the systolic pressure.

To keep the natural frequency as high as possible, the tubing should be wide bore, short, and rigid (little compliance). The number of stopcocks should be kept to a minimum as they have a relatively small lumen and tend to trap and hold small air bubbles. Large air bubbles cause damping of the system, whereas small air bubbles decrease the natural frequency of the system causing ringing. Occasionally it is necessary to use long extension tubing for monitoring patients in the operating room. The user must realize this introduces a considerable amount of ringing and the systolic overshoot may be tremendous. In such cases the most accurate pressure is the mean pressure.

Calibration of the pressure transducer first requires "zeroing" with reference to atmospheric pressure. This should be done when the tubing and transducer are filled with fluid and are free of air bubbles. Most

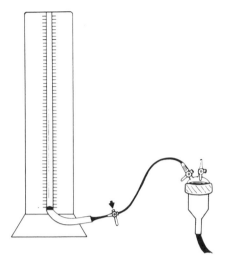

FIG. 14. Use of mercury manometer to verify calibration of blood pressure transducer. The mercury column is raised to the desired level by injecting fluid into the system (**arrow**). Blood pressure display should equal height of the column (mmHg).

monitoring kits have a stopcock attached, or very close, to the transducer dome. This stopcock should be opened so the transducer diaphragm is exposed to atmospheric pressure. After verifying that the transducer cable is properly attached to the physiologic monitor, the amplifier should be adjusted so the monitor reads "O". Most modern amplifiers designed for clinical monitoring have simplified controls for establishing a zero-pressure baseline and calibration. Monitors that use these simplified controls for calibration should be verified by using a mercury manometer. (Fig. 14). The system is satisfactory if high pressures are accurate within 5% and low pressures within 10%. It is important to verify that the baseline does not wander; e.g., when the stopcock used for zeroing is opened to air, the monitor should continuously display "0".

When the patient's artery has been cannulated and the catheter is connected to the pressure monitoring system, adjust the level of the transducer so the meniscus in the stopcock used for zeroing is at the level of the left ventricle. In the supine patient this corresponds to the mid-axillary line. If the patient is moved up or down with respect to the transducer, the pressure measured will then change. If the patient is higher than the transducer, then the pressure will equal that of the patient plus that exerted by the column of fluid in the tubing. If the patient is lower, the opposite is seen.

Equipment for Invasive Monitoring

1. A physiologic monitor with an attached pressure transducer.
2. Monitoring kit containing high pressure tubing, stopcocks, connec-

tors, caps, transducer dome, IV tubing, and high-pressure/low flow device.
3. 500 ml bag of saline with 500 units of heparin (one unit/ml).
4. Pressure bag to put the heparinized saline under 300 mmHg pressure.
5. Suitable arterial catheter, 24 gauge to 20 gauge.
6. Iodophore or antibiotic ointment to be placed at catheterization site.
7. Adhesive tape, preferably waterproof type.

Arterial pressure wave. As the arterial pressure pulse wave passes from the root of the aorta to the periphery, its form undergoes several changes (Fig. 15). These transformations are complex and poorly understood, although most of the changes are explained by reflected waves adding or subtracting from the incident wave. It is thought that most of the reflection occurs at the artery-arterial junction. As the pressure wave travels to the extremities, it becomes steeper and the systolic pressure becomes higher. In general, the further into the periphery blood pressure is measured, the narrower the waveform appears; the systolic pressure becomes higher and the diastolic pressure is lower. The mean pressure, however, remains relatively the same.

Noninvasive Blood Pressure Monitoring

Every noninvasive method of measuring blood pressure involves compressing an artery. There are three distinct manual (or nonautomatic) methods:

1. Pulse Palpation. An inflatable cuff is placed around a leg or arm and inflated until the cuff exerts a pressure on the limb that is greater than that in the major artery within the limb. This stops (occludes) blood flow in the artery and the palpable pulse in the artery distal to the cuff disappears. If the cuff then is slowly deflated, the pulse can be felt again when cuff pressure falls below the heart's maximum pulse pressure. This is the systolic pressure and is read from a manometer attached to the cuff. The manometer needle will bounce with each pulse until the pressure on the artery reaches the approximate diastolic valve. Below that pressure, the needle will fall without bouncing. This technique is almost always used on the upper arm where the brachial artery is occluded and the radial artery is palpated at the wrist. While requiring a minimum of equipment, pulse palpation is obviously of minimal accuracy, especially for diastolic pressure, as it depends on sensitive palpation of the radial artery, careful reading of the manometer, and a slow, consistent deflation technique (Fig. 16). Beyond its functional limitations, monitoring blood pressure by palpation is impractical for the anesthesiologist.
2. Doppler (ultrasound) Detection. As the pulse palpation method is lim-

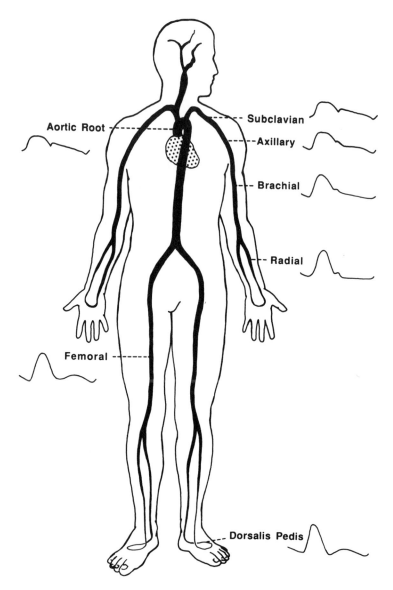

FIG. 15. Shape of the arterial pressure pulse wave as it appears when recorded at different points of the arterial system.

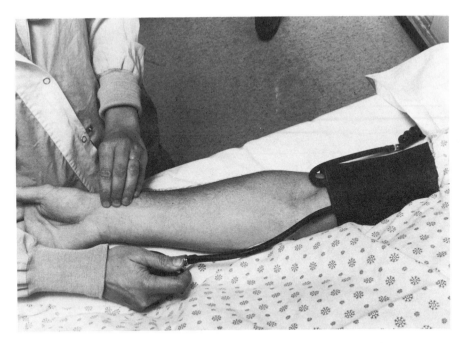

FIG. 16. Determining blood pressure by pulse palpation. Wall-mounted mercury manometer is connected to cuff.

ited in part by reliance on human tactile perceptions, it can be improved slightly by using a more sensitive detector of blood flow. Small noninvasive ultrasound (Doppler) probes are available to serve this need. Doppler detectors (discussed later in this chapter) provide an audio indication of flow in vessels. By deflating the cuff until the first indication of a pulse on the Doppler device, systolic pressure can be determined more accurately (Fig. 17). However, the point at which the diastolic pressure is reached is indicated by a subtle and qualitative change in the Doppler tone, and the diastolic value is only approximated. This technique can be an acceptable alternative to conventional methods in situations where pressure values are unusually low, or when blood pressure must be obtained from a leg rather than from an arm.

3. Auscultation (Method of Riva-Rocci). This method, the most familiar in any clinical setting, was first described by Scipione Riva-Rocci around 1900. An occlusive cuff is used as described above; however, changes in blood flow are detected using Korotkoff sounds through a conventional stethoscope placed in close proximity to an artery distal (downstream) from the occluding cuff. These sounds are distinctive, high-pitched sounds created by turbulent blood flow, and they occur

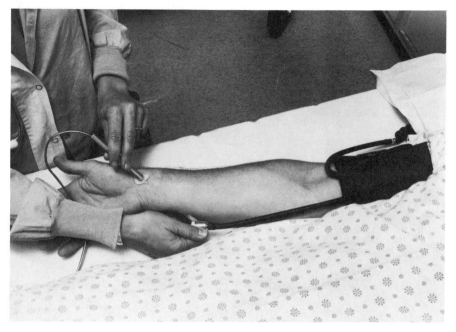

FIG. 17. Blood pressure by Doppler detection. Note use of ultrasound gel at the probe.

at each pulse. The manometer reading when the first Korotkoff sound is heard during cuff deflation indicates systolic pressure. As the cuff is deflated further, pressure equal to the diastolic value is reached; at this point the artery is no longer deformed by the cuff, and therefore blood flow is no longer turbulent. At this pressure Korotkoff sounds change from high-pitched to low-pitched, muffled signals. The conventional technique is to occlude the brachial artery at the upper arm, and auscultate (listen for) sounds at the same artery just below the elbow (Fig. 18). In monitoring for anesthesia, the stethoscope may be one of several styles designed for repetitive monitoring; these are secured to the arm or under the blood pressure cuff.

The American Heart Association standard for the inflatable bladder of the blood pressure cuff to cover is approximately 80% of the circumference of the arm, and on cuff deflation, the pressure should decrease at 2 or 3 mm Hg per second. If a cuff is too small for the patient's arm, falsely elevated pressures can be measured. If the cuff is deflated too rapidly, the first Korotkoff sound will be heard at a falsely low value.

Manual blood pressure equipment is relatively simple, but it is easily abused. Bladders in cuffs will deteriorate over time and develop small

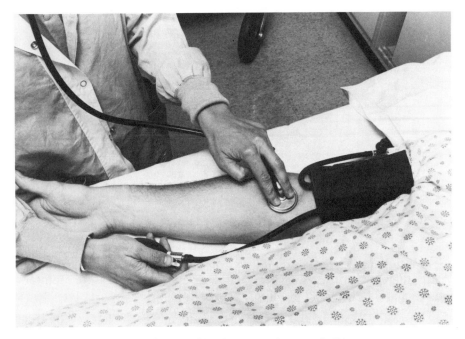

FIG. 18. Blood pressure by auscultation.

pinhole leaks; the bladders are easily replaced. A newer type of cuff, which incorporates the bladder into the cuff design, is lighter and easier to clean, but must be discarded if found to leak. In either case, one must check for suspected leaks by submerging the partially inflated bladder/cuff in water while watching for a trail of air bubbles. Dust or residue may cause the bleed valve and check valve of inflation bulbs to stick. These can be restored to function by flushing with alcohol or other solvents, then blowing dry. The blood pressure manometer is the weak point in most systems; with little variation, it consists of a semirigid closed chamber connected to the source of pressure (Fig. 19). As pressure is applied to the interior of the chamber, the manometer distends or bulges on one side, where a mechanical arrangement of levers or a gear train causes a needle to rotate. The range for this application is set at 0 to 300 mmHg, and is calibrated at the factory. Manometers do not survive abuse very well; a fall to the floor or severe impact anywhere can jam the mechanical linkage so the meter will not operate at all. General abuse can cause the meter to become inaccurate at the high or low ends of its scale, which can result in misleading blood pressure readings. Ideally, manometers should be checked against a mercury manometer annually or whenever they are suspected of being inaccurate.

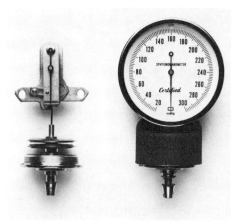

FIG. 19. Internal and external views of standard aneroid manometer. The semi-rigid chamber can be seen as two thin discs above the threaded mount (**left**). As pressure in these discs increases, they force the rod upward, activating a gear-train that causes the needle to rotate clockwise.

Automated methods of noninvasive blood pressure measurement. Currently there are at least fourteen models of automatic pressure monitors on the market. They fall into four distinct categories:

1. Ultrasonic. Among the first units produced in the late 1960s, one model uses a version of doppler detection of pulses more elegant than the one previously described. However, rather than detecting actual blood flow at an artery distal to the cuff, a sensor detects the motion of the arterial wall when it first "snaps" open as systolic pressure is reached. The wall motion continues until the decreasing cuff pressure reaches diastolic pressure, at which point the individual pulses no longer cause arterial wall movement. The Doppler crystals, located directly under the cuff, detect the first and last vessel wall motions; the associated electronics interpret these at the systolic and diastolic values, respectively. In the early model, the device used two mercury column manometers inflated to a preset value with each measurement. The cuff (and the connected manometers) were depressurized slowly; when the systolic was detected, the falling left column of mercury was stopped, as did the right column at the diastolic (Fig. 20). Later models replaced the mercury columns with digital meters.

    This technique remains functional, but as it depends on the detection of very small amounts of tissue motion, it is subject to interference from limb motion.

2. Oscillometry. This technique also uses an occlusive cuff. However, the sensors are transducers which detect pressure oscillations within the air bladder of the cuff or within the monitor box. The undulating vessel under the cuff conveys slight pressure waves through soft tissue and into the air within the cuff itself. The magnitude of these waves, or oscillations, serves as the indicator of systolic and mean pressures (diastolic pressure is calculated). (Fig. 20).

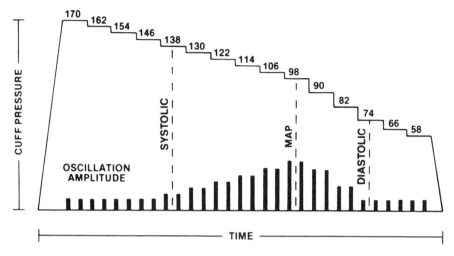

FIG. 20. Oscillometric detection of blood pressure. As pressure is incrementally decreased in the cuff, pressure waves are detected within the cuff and displayed as shown here. (Courtesy Critikon, Inc.; Copyright, 1986. Tampa, FL.)

Most of the automated BP monitors available today use the oscillometric technique. Since the cuff also serves as the detector of vessel motion, these units require no additional sensors. Detection of vessel oscillations, unfortunately, is more difficult at lower blood pressures; and it is at these lower values where accuracy is most important and where this technique may fail.

3. Auscultatory. Auscultatory models use the original concept of listening for Korotkoff sounds, but they do this electronically. Two acoustic sensors (essentially, tuned microphones) are incorporated into the cuff (Fig. 21). One, facing the limb, is sensitive to the higher frequencies characteristic of the turbulent blood flow at the systolic point. The other, facing into the air bag of the cuff, senses the lower pitches of the Korotkoff sounds at the diastolic point. By correlating cuff pressure and filtered signals from the two sensors, the electronics determine and display the values. This method is fairly consistent, but tends to be less practical than oscillometric devices.

In order to obtain more consistent readings from patients with unusually low pressures or varying heart rates, several models use both electronic auscultation and oscillometry; if one detection mode fails or is extraneous, the electronics accept the values from the other mode.

General comments regarding blood pressure cuffs. Most difficulties associated with the use of noninvasive BP monitors relate to the cuff. If the cuff has a leak, the device usually will not determine a value (the pump will continue to attempt to reach the usual starting pressure

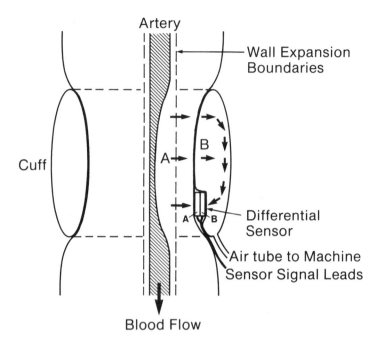

FIG. 21. Automated auscultatory detection of blood pressure. Differential sensor detects hi-pitched Korotkoff sounds at opening snap of vessel (**A**), and low-pitched sounds at diastolic point (**B**). (Courtesy Kendall Corp. Mansfield, MA.)

of 160 or 180 mmHg, then quit after several cycles). If the tubing to the cuff is pinched or kinked, the device will also detect the problem and quit. The cuff must be the proper size for the limb; oversized cuffs will render inaccurate readings and too small a cuff will pull loose upon inflation. The air should be squeezed out of the cuff before application. Secure the limb so it will be "quiet" during measurements; surgical personnel may bump BP cuffs sufficiently to cause the device to default. Most models reliably reject extraneous signals ("artifact"), but they can be deceived.

Many models have diagnostic codes which are displayed in the event of failure; interpret these if they are displayed and make appropriate corrections. Although generally consistent and reliable, these devices should be calibrated annually, or immediately, if reliability is in doubt.

4. Photoplethysmography. This category involves the use of a light source to detect blood flow.

A small cuff which includes the infrared emitter and detector is placed around the end of a finger and inflated until its pressure (as indicated by a specific light signal) is equal to that in the digital arteries (Figs. 22A,B). The arteries are said to be "unloaded", that is, the

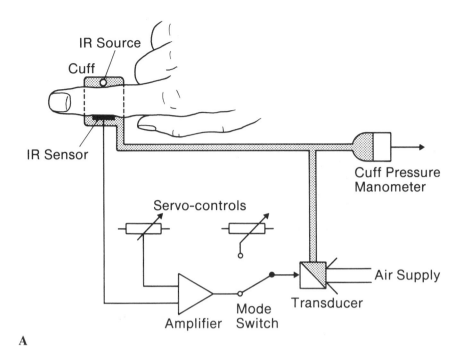

A

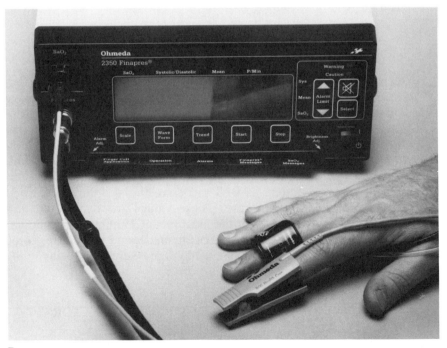

B

FIG. 22. A. Diagram of automated servo-controller photoplethysmograph blood pressure monitor. **B.** Ohmeda 2350 Finapres® photoplethysmographic blood pressure monitor. (Reprinted with permission from J.C., Dorlas, et al. (1985): *Anesthesiology.* Lippincott, Philadelphia.) (*Figure continues.*)

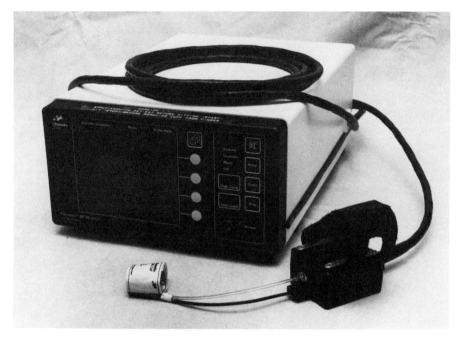

FIG. 22 (*Continued*)   **C.** Early model of Ohmeda monitor.

external pressure equals their internal, "loaded", pressure. The cuff pressure now is continually adjusted up or down by a very responsive pump, so that the light signal remains unchanged as the cuff pressure is varied in step with the pressure in the arteries. Thus, the dynamically changing cuff pressure "tracks" the arterial pressure almost instantaneously and effectively copies the arterial pressure waveform. Microprocessor-based electronics display the cuff pressure waveform graphically on a monitor, as well as derive the systolic, mean, and diastolic values, and heart rate. These values are also stored in a memory to display trends over the most recent 15 minutes to 8 hours. Refinements to the system are still being made, and it promises to be a major improvement in noninvasive blood pressure monitoring in the operating room.

ULTRASOUND (DOPPLER) BLOOD FLOW DETECTORS

The term "ultrasound" refers to acoustic wave energy (*not* radio waves) whose frequencies are above the range of human hearing. Ultrasound waves behave much like light waves in that they are *reflected* from surfaces; they are *refracted* (i.e., change angle of direction) when they pass into a material or different density; and they change frequency when reflected by a moving object. This last feature, known as Doppler shift, is classically recognized in the changing pitch of a train whistle as the train approaches and passes. The Doppler shift phenomenon has been known for decades, but only in the mid 1960s did it become practical to apply in clinical settings. In diagnostic work, and during or immediately after surgery, it is very useful to have a means of detecting blood flow in arterial vessels. The majority of the ultrasound devices are designed for transcutaneous use (i.e., they detect across skin) (Fig. 23). However, the returning signal, because of Doppler shift, will be slightly offset from the original signal. The blood components are in motion and cause the frequency to shift in proportion to their average speed. The greater their speed, the greater the difference between the transmitted and received frequencies. This difference signal, which is within the range of human hearing, can be separated by the electronics and amplified to hear on a speaker or headset, or processed further and recorded. If the flow in the vessel is smooth and nonturbulent (as in a vein), the Doppler signal heard will be a smooth, unchanging hiss or roar. In the more typical case of detecting flow in an artery, the audio signal is a distinctive, periodic swishing sound which identifies the pulsatile flow of arterial blood. The higher the audio frequency shift, the greater the motion being detected. A relatively loud "swishing" at one artery indicates a more dynamic blood flow than a lower-volume, lower-frequency "swooshing" report at another.

Use of Doppler shift depends primarily on reflection of the signal by the formed elements in blood (and to a much smaller extent, the motion of the vessel walls). If the vessel transports only liquid without cells or particles (e.g., water or saline), there is no audible Doppler shift.

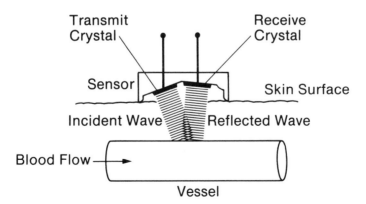

FIG. 23. Diagram of ultrasound (Doppler) detection of blood flow. (Reprinted with permission from J. Carr and J. Brown (1981): *Introduction to Biomedical Equipment Technology,* 1st ed. John Wiley & Sons, Inc., New York.)

Transcutaneous ultrasound is both art and science as it provides qualitative, but not quantitative, information. The sounds produced must be interpreted and compared, but do not provide actual blood flow data in liters/min. In the vascular diagnostic laboratory, more sophisticated doppler devices which determine blood flow are in routine use.

The frequency used by the Doppler device is determined mainly by the size and depth of the vessels under scrutiny; larger, deeper vessels require a frequency range of 2 to 4 MHz, while smaller peripheral vessels require frequencies of 9 to 10 MHz. In most models the transmit and receive crystals are fabricated into one sensing probe or disc which connects to the remaining electronics in a portable box (Fig. 24). Since ultrasound is refracted when passing through different media, it is essential to provide a path for the signal from sensor to skin which is about the same density as the patient's soft tissue. Air pockets or bubbles cannot be allowed in the path of the signal. For this reason, a small amount of "coupling medium" must always be applied at the sensor face. This is a water-based gel or cream available from the device's manufacturer, formulated specifically for this purpose. In its absence, any viscous lubricating jellies commonly found in clinical settings can be used, but with

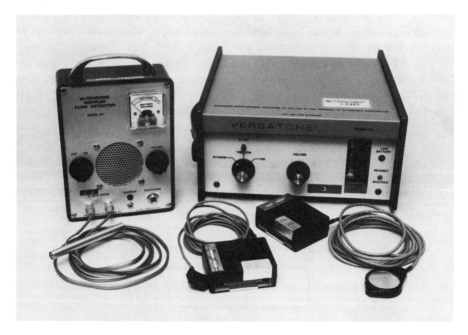

FIG. 24. Two standard portable doppler units. Model (**left**) uses a 9.2 MHz probe for smaller, peripheral vessels. Unit (**right**) accepts several probes; 10 MHz and 4 MHz probes shown here.

less benefit. Note that there should be a relatively acute angle between the sensor and the vessel axis; if the angle is 90° (i.e., if the signal passes at a right angle to the vessel), there will be little or no doppler shift detected (Fig. 25). In the case of the higher-frequency "pencil" type probes, rotating the probe also will help provide an optimized signal. Square or disc-shaped sensors must be secured in place after the best signal output is found by careful trial-and-error. Use a generous amount of interface gel to secure the sensor with a tenacious type of adhesive tape. This is especially important during continuous doppler monitoring of the right side of the heart to detect air emboli during surgeries in which there is a risk of entraining air into the venous system (Fig. 26). The passage of this air can be detected by the doppler signal as a distinctive, high-frequency rattle, which enables the physician to intervene.

Doppler equipment tends to be relatively maintenance free, except for routine cleaning and inspection after each use. Residual interface gel should be rinsed off the sensor immediately after use and before the gel dries; a cotton-tip applicator may be necessary to clear residual gel from the recesses of some designs. The greatest liability of any model is its sensor. The crystal elements are fragile and will not tolerate abusive

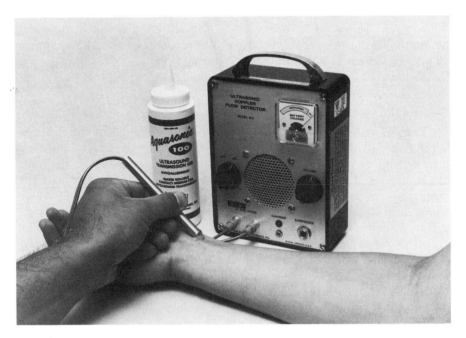

FIG. 25. Use of a peripheral Doppler probe. Note angle of probe and use of ultrasound gel.

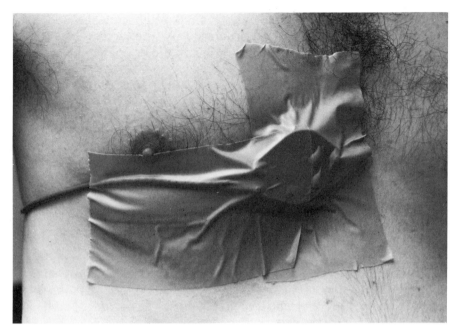

FIG. 26. Low-frequency Doppler sensor secured to patient's chest for detection of air bubbles in major venous blood vessels.

handing; Once cracked, a crystal will not resonate. The gel and sensor should be stored with the unit.

CENTRAL VENOUS PRESSURE MONITORING

Clinicians often place a catheter into the right atrium of the heart as another IV site and as a site for pressure monitoring. Access to this area may be from any of several peripheral locations. In anesthesia, the most common sites are the internal jugular vein, subclavian vein, or one of the large veins in the arm (basilic, median cephalic). Depending on which site is used, it takes a fairly long catheter to reach the right atrium (e.g., a 5 to 8 inch catheter is used for the internal jugular and subclavian veins). Normal pressure in the right atrium is from 0 mmHg to 7 mmHg, and represents what is known as preload, or the amount of volume available to the right side of the heart. Conversely, afterload is the term used to describe the work the left ventricle must do to eject blood. Not only is central venous pressure a monitor of preload, but it may also reflect right and left ventricular dysfunction.

There is a classic CVP waveform that may be used clinically. In the operating room it is often convenient to connect the central line to a water manometer. When a water manometer is used, the units of pressure are recorded in cm/H_2O, and not mmHg. The ratio of the specific gravity of mercury and water is 13.6 : 1; therefore, 1 cm/H_2O = 1.36 mmHg. It is important to note this difference because many workers report numbers without the corresponding units, leaving room for error. At low pressures, the difference between cm/H_2O and mmHg is small, but at higher pressures it becomes very significant. The CVP changes with respiration; the desired pressure is that obtained at the end of exhalation. Also, patients on a ventilator and receiving PEEP (positive-end-expiratory-pressure) should be disconnected briefly in order to avoid falsely high values.

If the CVP is being measured with a pressure transducer, set the monitor so it is displaying the mean pressure. If it is desirable to see the waveform, it is best to use a monitor that allows the user to adjust the pressure scale. As CVP is a low pressure with the monitor set to the lowest scale, the amplitude of the waveforms will be increased so it is easily recognized. Many patients will have an art-line in place and connected to a transducer when the decision to monitor the CVP is announced. If the clinician wants to measure the CVP only intermittently, an IV extension line can be attached to the central-line and connected to a fitting on the stopcock. This fitting already exists on the art-line set-up and may require the use of a male-male adapter. High-pressure tubing is not required for the connection between the transducer and the central line, because only mean pressure which is not altered by compliant tubing is measured. This set-up requires the use of only one transducer and allows for rapid, accurate measurement of CVP by merely turning the direction of the stopcock.

CARDIAC OUTPUT MONITORING

Cardiac output is the volume of blood flowing in the ascending aorta in one minute. A normal range for cardiac output in a resting adult is 4 to 6 liters/min. For many years, the only technique for determining output was the modified Fick method, in which a known quantity of dye was injected into a major vessel as it entered the right heart; a series of blood samples were then taken from a small artery (e.g., the brachial or radial arteries). The dye (cardio-green) was detected in the blood samples by a densitometer, and a curve was generated by plotting dye levels against time. As we know the amount of dye initially injected and the time required for all dye to pass, the area under the curve can be interpreted as the cardiac output. This dye dilution method is accurate and lends itself to research studies, but is impractical in the patient care setting.

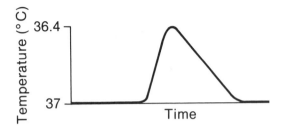

FIG. 27. Idealized shift in temperature of pulmonary artery after injection of cold solution. Note that the temperature scale is inverted. (Reprinted with permission from J. S. Gravenstein and D. A. Paulus (1982): *Monitoring Practice in Anesthesia*, 1st ed. Lippincott, Philadelphia, PA.)

A more clinically practical method became possible with the widespread use of pulmonary artery catheters. In one version of the pulmonary artery catheter, a thermistor-type sensor measures the temperature of the blood. By injecting a known amount of relatively cold solution through a small port on the catheter (about 26 cm upstream from the thermistor), the downward temperature shift of the blood will be detected, producing a curve virtually identical to that in the dye dilution technique (Fig. 27). In the thermodilution method, cardiac output is determined by the volume of cold injectate (usually 10 cc); the initial temperatures of the blood and of the injectate (typically 37°C and 0°C); and the area under the thermodilution curve. The determination is made by any of several microprocessor-based computers on the market which connect to the catheter (Fig. 28). The thermodilution technique compares well with the dye dilution method, and is much more practical in the OR and intensive care unit. However, both methods are invasive. They require the use of indwelling catheters at or near the heart and carry the risks associated with their placement.

A system has been on the market recently which takes advantage of advanced ultrasound (doppler) technology to determine cardiac output relatively noninvasively (Fig. 29). In the system in clinical use, a probe whose tip contains 2.5 MHz Doppler transducer crystals is advanced into the esophagus. With cautious trial-and-error positioning, the transducer is oriented to sense blood flow in the descending aorta, which is immediately adjacent the esophagus (Fig. 30a). With a slight correction factor, the blood flow can approximate the flow in the ascending aorta, and therefore the true cardiac output. The probe is connected to its dedicated computer-monitor which must know the diameter of the patient's aorta; this can be entered directly (if known from a direct determination), or it can be derived by the computer if the patient's sex, age, height, and weight are known. Since cardiac output is known, the monitor can also derive cardiac index (cardiac output/body surface area) and approximate systemic vascular resistance. The values displayed by the monitor are averaged and updated every 15 seconds. Before continuous monitoring, the system requires an initial value of cardiac output to use as a refer-

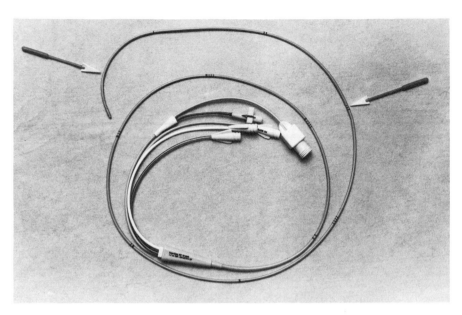

FIG. 28. Typical 3-lumen pulmonary artery catheter. **Left arrow** indicates location of thermistor sensor; **right arrow** shows port from which injectate enters the blood stream.

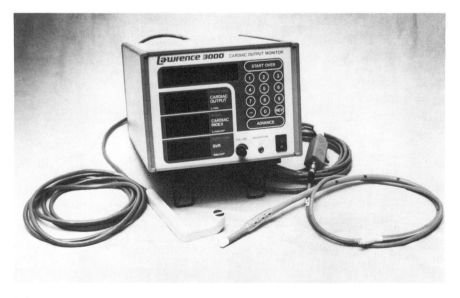

FIG. 29. Current noninvasive cardiac output monitor. (Courtesy Lawrence Medical Corp., Camarillo, CA.)

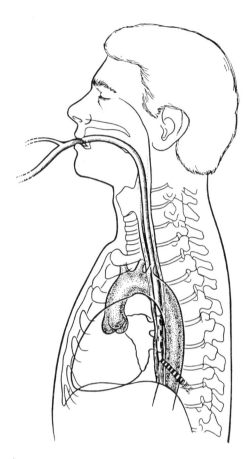

FIG. 30. A. Placement of a Doppler probe in the esophagus, showing sensor oriented toward the aorta (shaded vessel). B. Suprasternal Doppler probe oriented toward the ascending aorta. Note that there is also a Doppler probe in the esophagus. (Courtesy Lawrence Medical Corp., Camarillo, CA.)

A

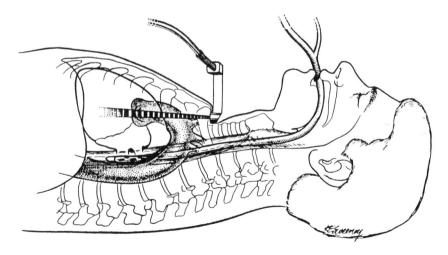

B

ence; in actual practice, this can be entered if known already, or determined by the use of a second ultrasound probe aimed downward at the ascending aorta from immediately above the sternum (Fig. 30b). This "suprasternal" probe can also be used for single determinations whenever indicated.

Management of the equipment is no different from that for transcutaneous Doppler devices, with particular respect to the (very expensive) probes. The esophageal probe should be cleaned and ETO-gas sterilized after each use.

Chapter 7

Respiratory Monitoring

END-TIDAL CARBON DIOXIDE MONITORS
(CAPNOMETERS AND CAPNOGRAPHS)

Monitoring carbon dioxide (CO_2) in a patient's breathing circuit during general anesthesia has become a standard of care. *Capnometry* refers to the measurement and numerical display of end-tidal CO_2; *capnography* is the recording of the CO_2 waveform in the breathing system. Information gained from such monitoring includes, but is not limited to, assurance that the endotracheal tube is correctly placed and that ventilation is adequate. Recall that CO_2, which is produced by the body during metabolism, is carried by the blood to the lungs where it is eliminated.

There are two categories of capnometers (Figs. 1A,B): (1) sensor within the ventilatory pathway and (2) sensor external to the ventilatory pathway. Both measure CO_2 by the same principle; that is, the absorption of infrared light by CO_2. An infrared light beam is projected through the gas sample, and the intensity of transmitted light is measured. There is an inverse relationship between the amount of CO_2 in the sample and the transmitted light intensity (Figs. 2A,B).

When sensors are to be placed in the ventilatory pathway, they are contained in hollow tubes that are placed in the patient's breathing system (Fig. 3). Gas movement past the sensor is caused by the patient's spontaneous breathing or by a ventilator. When the sensor is remote from the patient's breathing system a pump, which is part of the capnometer, sucks gas for analysis from the patient's breathing system, and delivers it via a sampling line to the sensor (Fig. 4). The rate of this gas sampling varies from 50 to 500 ml/min. After passing through the measuring chamber, the gas is exhausted through an output port where it may be scavenged to a disposal system. In infants and small children, end-tidal CO_2 is most accurately measured from sampling catheters placed at the distal tip of the endotracheal tube. Distal-sampling catheters and adaptor elbows are available commercially from Dryden Corporation, Indianapolis, Ind.

One of the more troublesome problems with the first generation of

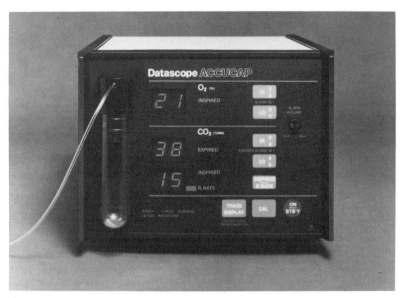

A

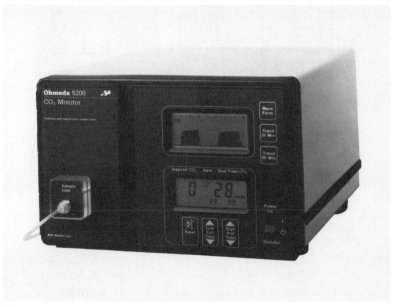

B

FIG. 1. Standard CO_2 monitors. **A.** Note that numerical values are displayed. "Trace Display" key enables the display of the CO_2 waveform on another monitor. (Courtesy Datascope Corporation, Paramus, NJ.) **B.** Upper display shows CO_2 waveform or can display a 20 or 60 minute trend of CO_2. Numerical values are displayed beneath the waveform. (Courtesy Ohmeda, The BOC Group, Inc., Madison, WI.)

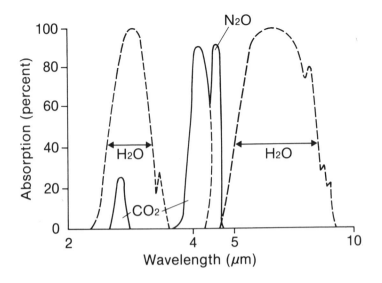

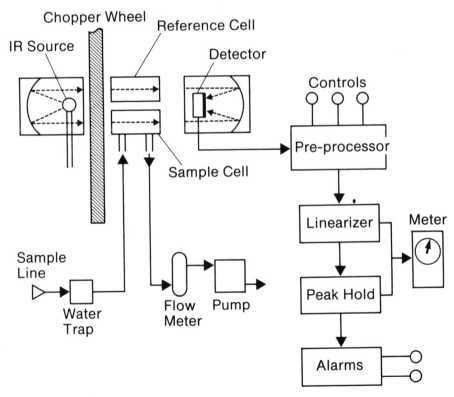

FIG. 2. **A.** Infrared absorption spectrum of CO_2, water (H_2O), and nitrous oxide (N_2O). Note the proximity of the CO_2 absorption peaks to the N_2O, and water peaks. (Reprinted with permission from: *Health Devices* (1986):286. Emergency Care Research Institute. Plymouth Meeting, PA.) **B.** Generalized schematic for the detection of CO_2 by infrared light. (Courtesy Instrumentation Laboratory, Fisher Scientific Company, Lexington, MA.)

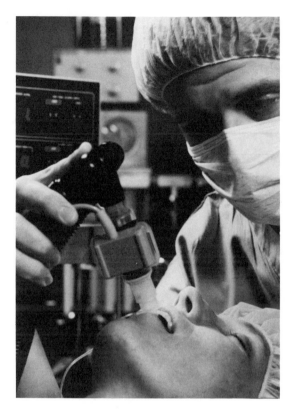

FIG. 3. "Mainstream" CO_2 sampling. IR source, reference, and chopper wheel are all located within the sensor shown here between the endotracheal tube and the patient breathing system (black tubing). (Reprinted with permission. Courtesy Hewlett-Packard Company, Palo Alto, CA.)

sidestream CO_2 analyzers was water accumulation in the sample system. The patient's exhaled gas mixture naturally contains water vapor at body temperature; when expired gas is drawn through the sample tube to the analyzer, the water cools and condenses within the tube. In short time, water droplets or secretions accumulate, occlude the tube, and may be drawn into the sample cell. Most manufacturers have addressed this problem with a very efficient trap or absorbent filter located at the monitor, where large amounts of water are removed without affecting the gas sample flow. Another solution is the use of a special sample tubing (Nafion) which allows water vapor to diffuse through the tubing wall. When sensors are placed in the ventilatory pathway, the device is heated to avoid water condensation. To avoid burns, it is important to prevent the sensor from touching the patient's skin.

The routine setup of earlier CO_2 monitors required several minutes of calibration. The necessity for accuracy in CO_2 values and because of the small range being measured, many units required the use of a calibration gas with which to adjust the upper end of the monitor's scale. Having confirmed a zero setting on room air and a high-end setting on calibration

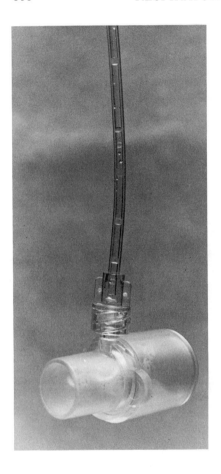

FIG. 4. CO_2 sampling device for remote CO_2 sensor. Note that it contains water introduced by condensation from the patient's exhaled gases. This water can prevent accurate CO_2 measurement.

gas (e.g., 5%), the unit should be ready. Current models of capnometers have internal zero and calibration.

The majority of problems occurring with CO_2 monitors with remote sensors involve the sample connector or tubing; droplets of water can occasionally migrate into the sample cell if the trap or filter fail, or if the sample flow rate is too high, or the tubing becomes kinked, pinched, or disconnected. Most of these problems do not occur when the sensor is in the airway. However, the sensor must be securely connected at the endotracheal tube; these sensors are relatively heavy and can bear down on the patient circuit, thereby risking disconnection, kinking of the endotracheal tube, and damage to the sensor.

Maintenance of capnometers includes washing the sensors. Indications and procedures for cleaning outlines in the manufacturer's manual should be consulted.

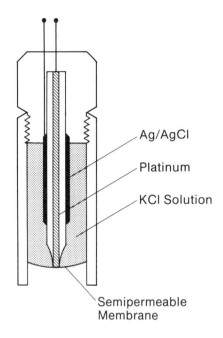

Ag/AgCl

Platinum

KCl Solution

Semipermeable
Membrane

FIG. 5. The Clark electrode as configured for oxygen monitors.

OXYGEN MONITORS

There are two types of oxygen analyzers in common use for anesthesia: the *polarographic* and the *fuel cell*. Both types of analyzers interpret the amount of oxygen in the sample in terms of electrical current or voltage. In the *polarographic* oxygen analyzer, the oxygen is detected in a two-part chemical reaction. With the assistance of a small voltage, oxygen combines with potassium chloride (KCl) to liberate a chloride ion (Cl^-). In the second reaction, the chloride ion combines with silver, and liberates electrons, thereby creating an electrical current. The amount of current created is proportional to the oxygen present. In most models, the current is converted to voltage and displayed on a meter at the analyzer. The chemical reactions (an "oxidation-reduction" reaction) take place in a small cartridge known as a Clark electrode, which is placed at the point of interest and connected to the electronics at a convenient location nearby (Fig. 5).

The oxygen sensing electrode is an expendable item (i.e., it has a limited lifetime) because the reactions taking place within it will eventually consume the potassium chloride (KCl) solution and the silver. The KCl solution can be replaced, but when the silver is depleted, the entire cartridge must be replaced. The membrane at the tip of the sensor is critical to the performance of the device: it allows oxygen to migrate while maintaining an interface with the KCl solution. If the membrane becomes loose or breaks, the sensor will fail.

The other oxygen analyzer also measures in terms of electrical energy, but does so by means of a *fuel cell*, a cartridge or cylinder in which a single chemical reaction continuously creates a small voltage (Fig. 6). Here the amount of available oxygen is proportional to the voltage created, but the relationship is not as linear as in the polarographic sensor. The voltage is displayed on a meter, calibrated in percent O_2.

In both types of analyzer, the expected lifetime of the sensor is dependent upon the amount of oxygen it is exposed to over time; manufacturers express life expectancy in O_2%-hours. Thus, a typical life expectancy for a polarographic cell may be 300,000 O_2%-hours between replenishments of the KCl solution. If the sensor is exposed to 50% O_2 each hour on average, this would represent 6,000 hours, or about 8 months. Fuel cell sensors operate continuously, without requiring a voltage (note that the polarographic sensor requires a voltage in its first reaction). The polarographic sensor will tolerate high levels of CO_2 and anesthetic agents without adverse effect on O_2 readings, but will not tolerate heavy condensation of water at its membrane. Fuel cells are unaffected by water.

In all cases, oxygen analyzers include either an analog meter or digital display of O_2 percent, a means for calibration of the meter, and an adjustable low-alarm which activates an audio signal (beeper or continuous tone) when the oxygen concentration falls below the alarm limit. Since patients, under no circumstances, should be delivered less than the 21%

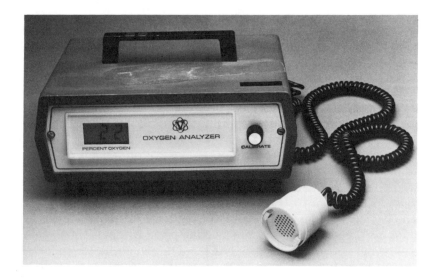

FIG. 6. Typical fuel-cell type O_2 sensor and monitor.

O_2 of the atmosphere, the low-alarm usually has a minimum set-point of around 20%. Many models offer a high-alarm setting as well.

The use of an oxygen analyzer generally has been taken as a standard of care in the anesthesia community; until replaced by other technologies, it will be an essential part of the anesthetic delivery system. It should not be overlooked or taken lightly in routine equipment maintenance or daily machine checks. Virtually all models are battery-operated (including fuel-cell types for the alarm circuits); batteries should be checked routinely, and replaced when indicated. Assured of adequate battery level, the unit should be checked for calibration at *two* points; checking the calibration at only one point does not insure accuracy. One must expose the sensor to room air and adjust the reading to 21%, if necessary, then expose the sensor to 100% of O_2 from the anesthesia machine's delivery port (2–4 L/min of 100% O_2) and ascertain a reading of 100% $\pm$ 3%. Failure to calibrate usually indicates the need to replenish or replace the sensor. The unit probably is defective if it will not calibrate well with fresh batteries and a new sensor.

PULSE-OXIMETERS

Oxygen saturation (SaO_2) is a measure of oxygenation in blood. Oxygen saturation is expressed as a percentage and is defined as the ratio of the oxyhemoglobin (HbO_2) to the total hemoglobin (Hb) present (i.e., hemoglobin with no O_2 molecules bound (Hbl), HbO_2, and other forms of Hb). The relationship between saturation and the partial pressure of the oxygen is, however, not linear; as the saturation drops below approximately 80%, the partial pressure of the oxygen drops dramatically, which means that it is effectively unable to support metabolism (Fig. 7). Any value of SaO_2 below 85%, therefore, is considered clinically dangerous.

In the late 1940s and early 1950s, a method was described to identify the levels of HbO_2 and Hb separately by virtue of their ability to absorb different wavelengths of light. Remember that light is a waveform phenomena, as are radio waves, and can be measured in terms of wave length at any frequency. HbO_2 absorbs light energy most at a wavelength of about 650 nanometers (nm) (1 nm = .000000001 meter); this appears to the eye as medium red light. Hb absorbs light energy in the infrared wavelengths of about 900 nm (Fig. 8). These two Hb components can be detected at different wavelengths and the SaO_2 can be derived by comparing them. Before the advent of microprocessors, this technique was difficult to apply in the clinical setting because interference from ambient light, motion of tissue, and the pulsations of arterial blood made the arterial saturation determination unreliable. In the early 1980s, these problems were overcome.

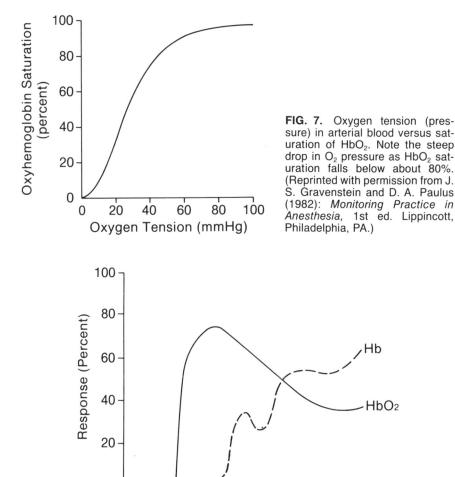

FIG. 7. Oxygen tension (pressure) in arterial blood versus saturation of HbO_2. Note the steep drop in O_2 pressure as HbO_2 saturation falls below about 80%. (Reprinted with permission from J. S. Gravenstein and D. A. Paulus (1982): *Monitoring Practice in Anesthesia,* 1st ed. Lippincott, Philadelphia, PA.)

FIG. 8. Infrared spectra of hemoglobin (Hb) and oxyhemoglobin (HbO_2).

In the standard model, a small sensor is placed on the end of a finger or toe, on the earlobe, on the foot (small infants), or across the bridge of the nose (Fig. 9). The sensor consists of two light-emitting diodes (LEDs) which emit light at the two wavelengths previously mentioned, and a "photodiode", a light sensitive transistor which produces a current proportionate to the light energy it detects. The LEDs are switched rapidly on and off (50 to 60 times/second) by the electronics, and the photodiode

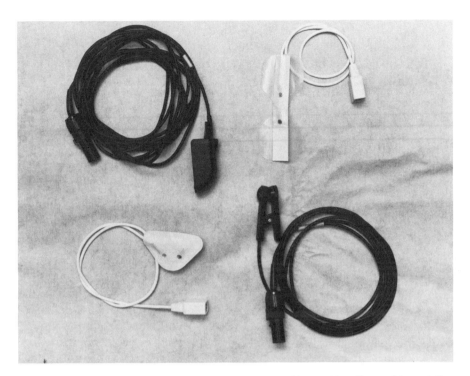

FIG. 9. Various sensors for current pulse-oximeters. **Above:** Non-disposable and disposable finger sensors **(left to right)**. **Below:** Sensors for the nose and earlobe **(left to right)**.

detects the levels of light which "survive" the passage through the blood supply of the soft tissue. The photodiode sends its current signals to the electronics, where they are interpreted in terms of Hb and HbO_2. After filtering out any extraneous values caused by motion at the sensor, the microprocessor calculates and displays the $SaO_2\%$ value. Changes in the signal strength because of the outside light or pressure on the soft tissue can also be compensated for by the electronics. Since the photodiode also sees changes in HbO_2 level due to the pulsations of arterial blood, the device can extract and display the pulse rate. The displayed values of SaO_2 and heart rate in most models are averaged over a 5 to 10 second period, so the values are not updated so often as to be distracting or spurious, yet respond quickly enough to indicate a clinically important trend. One model offers a choice of 6 second or 3 second averages. Some models provide true "trending" of the data by displaying the SaO_2 values as a graph over the most recent 20 or 60 minutes (Fig. 10).

As with almost all monitors for clinical use, pulse-oximeters include adjustable alarms for the variables being monitored. As they are micro-

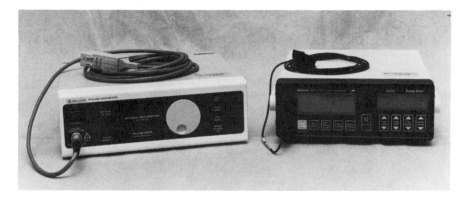

FIG. 10. Two current models of pulse-oximeter.

processor-based, the alarm settings are preset at generally accepted values of SaO_2 and pulse rate ("default" settings); typically a low SaO_2 alarm point of 85% and low pulse rate of 50 beats/minute. High SaO_2 and rate alarm points usually can be adjusted, or all alarms can be defeated. Adjustable audio tones for pulse and alarm violation are almost universal. One manufacturer's unit decreases its audio pitch with decreased SaO_2 values. Most models provide an output connector in the unit's back to enable users to record data on another device, or to communicate the data to other monitors.

Technical support required for pulse oximeters is minimal; the sensor, whether reusable or disposable, requires no replenishment of expendable material, and the monitor requires no on-site calibration. Most are battery operated with line-powered rechargeable batteries; failure of the battery supply is indicated at the display, and the unit will usually shut down rather than give erroneous data. The weak point of the system is the sensor-to-patient interface: if the sensor is poorly positioned or the ambient light too direct, the monitor will not receive readable signals. Some clinicians report better results with the finger or nose sensors than for the earlobe; the temperature or size of the earlobe may be factors. Some units have been said to be more sensitive than others to skin pigmentation, but revisions in the electronics have apparently increased the signal strength to compensate for lower light detection when necessary. There have been reports of one model giving acceptable, but inaccurate, SaO_2 readings when used in the presence of a specific model of surgical light. While the manufacturer has addressed this problem, it is a good practice wherever possible, to cover or "hide" the sensor from direct lighting. Other than awareness of these problems, users should routinely inspect the wire and connectors of the sensor; some tend to be easily frayed or cracked.

MULTIPLE GAS ANALYZERS

Multiple gas analysis based on infra-red absorption, mass spectrometry, or Raman spectroscopy is becoming increasingly common in the operating room to monitor the composition of the patient's inhaled and exhaled gas. These multiple gas monitors may be dedicated to one patient or they may be part of a shared system that serves a large number of operating rooms. These systems may measure up to eight gases (e.g., O_2, CO_2, N_2O, nitrogen, halothane, enflurane, isoflurane, helium). Multiple gas analysis is a rapidly evolving area. Therefore, we have elected not to discuss it in detail. A good introduction to the subject can be found in *Capnography in the Operating Room* by S. May, et al., listed in the Bibliography.

Chapter 8

Other Monitors and STAT Lab

TEMPERATURE MONITORS

Body temperature is routinely monitored throughout surgical procedures; all thermometers used for this purpose are electronic. Traditional mercury-in-glass thermometers are difficult to read and present a hazard in the OR. "Liquid-crystal" types of thermometers usually are thin plastic adhesive membranes that change color within a limited range of temperatures. They are difficult to read and have a poor response time, and therefore have never been well accepted for clinical applications. On the other hand, electronic thermometry provides good sensitivity, fast response to change, displays that can be read from a distance, and a variety of sensor locations on or in the body.

There are two types of electronic thermometers in common use today: *thermistor* and *thermocouple*. Both may appear physically similar, but they determine temperature differently. In the thermistor variety, the sensor consists of a material whose electrical resistance changes with change in temperature. This resistor is one of four resistors in a four-sided circuit which has a constant voltage applied at two points (Fig. 1). As the temperature at the sensing resistor changes, its resistance changes, causing the applied voltage to change. This "output voltage" is amplified and displayed on a meter or a digital display as temperature. The thermocouple type device takes advantage of the fact that a very small voltage is created at the junction of two dissimilar metals (e.g., copper and platinum). If this sensing junction is placed at the point of interest and its voltage compared with that of another junction whose temperature remains constant (the "reference" junction), the voltage difference between these two junctions can be amplified and interpreted as the temperature at the sensing point (Fig. 2). With both types of electronic thermometry there are limitations due to nonlinearity (i.e., the output voltages do not change in equal amounts at all temperature ranges). All of the devices, therefore, include circuitry which adequately compensates for this problem within the range of body temperatures.

Virtually all temperature monitors can display the temperature in Cel-

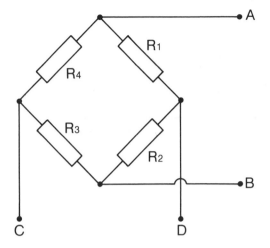

FIG. 1. Schematic of the resistance bridge used in thermistor-type thermometers (the "Wheatstone Bridge"). Constant voltage is applied between to A and B and voltage across C and D is measured. If the resistance of one element (e.g., R3) changes with temperature, voltage across C and D will change in proportion to the resistance (and hence temperature) change. When such circuitry is used for temperature monitoring, one of the resistors is the temperature sensor applied to the patient and the meter connected to C and D is calibrated in temperature units (i.e., volts are converted to temperature).

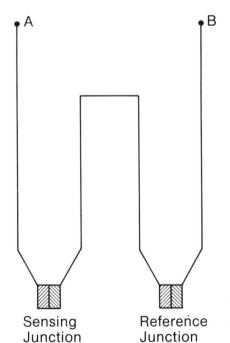

Sensing
Junction

Reference
Junction

FIG. 2. Schematic of the thermocouple type thermometer. The sensing junction is at the patient, the reference junction within the monitor. The signal processing and display circuitry is connected to A and B.

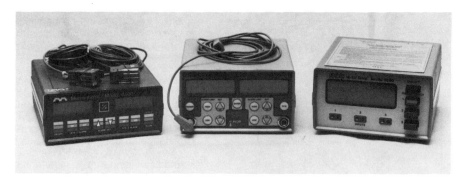

FIG. 3. Three standard electronic thermometers used in anesthesia. The Mon-a-therm **(left)** and RSP **(center)** devices have two temperature displays. The NCC device **(right)** has a single display. Temperatures detected from any one of three sensors can be selected by pushing the appropriate button.

sius (centigrade) or Fahrenheit scales, although Celsius is the standard for clinical work. The majority of these units display in digital format, rather than with meter movement. Many are dual units; effectively two separate thermometers in one box (Fig. 3). Most multi-function OR monitors include thermometry among their many functions, which helps reduce the number of devices in the anesthesiologist's work area.

Where the temperature sensor is placed on the patient remains a compromise between convenience and accuracy; skin sensors are easily applied, but skin temperature is often not a good indicator of the "core" temperature (i.e., temperature within the body). Placing a small sensing probe rectally gives a true core temperature, but is inconvenient in most cases. With the concern for malignant hyperthermia (rapid increase in body temperature, triggered by anesthetic drug, that may be fatal), some anesthesiologists believe that the large muscles of the thigh should be monitored by a skin sensor. Another approach is to use a sensor inserted in the ear canal, although this has resulted in some patient injuries. The most common approach to measuring temperature during general anesthesia is to use an esophageal stethoscope with a temperature sensor (Fig. 4). While temperature measured may be cooler than true core temperature, it is considered a good indicator of trends and is convenient to obtain.

The majority of sensors in use today are single-use disposables. The usual arguments for and against disposables apply here as they do elsewhere: disposables are time-saving and add a margin of assurance of sterility, but they cost more and waste resources.

Thermometry monitors require little maintenance beyond routine cleaning and inspection. Most are battery operated. Battery exhaustion is usually indicated at the display, and battery replacement can easily be

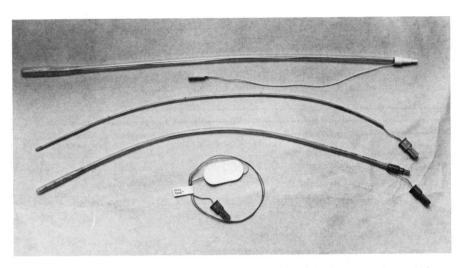

FIG. 4. Various disposable thermometer sensors. Thermistor-type: esophageal; thermocouple-type: rectal probe, esophageal, and skin. (**top to bottom, respectively**).

done. Sensors, reusable or disposable, occasionally fail, but the failure is usually extreme and obvious. In the event of any question of device failure, have the unit checked.

A third type of electronic thermometer has been introduced which measures temperature by detecting the infrared-wavelength energy emitted by any surface. These models are designed for measuring temperature at the tympanic membrane in the ear canal. Temperatures recorded in this manner compare well with core temperature. They are intended for individual readings with a hand-held probe, rather than for continuous monitoring by a secured sensor. It is yet to be determined if infrared thermometry lends itself to anesthesiology.

CONTROLLING THE PATIENT'S TEMPERATURE

Generally, positive steps are required to keep a patient's body temperature from falling during surgery. In the typical course of a surgical experience, the patient begins with no more protection from room temperature than a hospital gown and one or two cotton blankets. These usually are removed in the operating room and are replaced with various arrays of surgical drapes, often paper, designed to repel micro-organisms rather than preserve heat. Additionally, the patient is almost universally infused with room temperature IV solutions. Furthermore, anesthetic agents impair body thermoregulation.

Thermal Barriers and Warming Blankets

There has been a gradual acceptance of metallized plastic "thermal barrier" drapes and head covers designed to be placed on the patient (ideally, before the patient is brought to the OR suite) before the sterile drapes are applied (Fig. 5). It is increasingly common to minimize heat loss during surgery by placing a "warming pad" under the patient. This pad has a network of coils through which warm water circulates; temperature of the water can be adjusted within safe limits. A water pad can also serve as a cooling blanket for specific cases, notably open heart procedures, where it is desirable to reduce the patient's temperature. Thus it is often labeled a "hypothermia/hyperthermia" system (Fig. 6). In the recovery room, infrared heat lamps are frequently used to raise and/or maintain body temperature.

Fluid Warmers

Infusing warm fluids into patients can also aid in maintaining body temperature. Many anesthesia personnel pre-warm bags or bottles of IV solutions in a solution warming cabinet or blanket warmer. In the 1950s, devices became commercially available to warm banked units of blood for transfusion; anesthesiologists were aware of the adverse effects of administering refrigerated blood (usually kept at 4°C), and the *blood warmer* became a routine accessory in cases where multiple units of blood were to be infused. Blood warmers are now used to warm IV solutions and volume expanders as well as whole blood; hence, they should more accurately be referred to as *fluid warmers*.

These devices can be divided into two categories based on the methods by which energy is transferred to the fluid being infused: in *water bath types,* the fluid is passed through a tube or coil which is immersed in warm water; in *dry heat types,* the coil or bag is held directly against a heated metal plate or cylinder (Fig. 7). In all cases, the path of the infused fluid must remain sterile. Virtually all warmers require the use of a single-use disposable fluid delivery set, which connects to the fluid bag or bottle on one end and terminates with a conventional Luer fitting at the patient end. In most models, care must be taken to avoid pinching the tubing or corners of the bag as it is installed in the warmer. All warmers use electrically driven heating elements similar to a kitchen toaster, and must be regulated to switch off at a certain temperature. The consequences of overheating infused fluids, especially whole blood, can be very serious, so fluid warmers usually have two or three stages of regulation. The American Association of Blood Bank's (AABB) standard for transfusion states that blood should not be delivered above 37°C. Most fluid warmers heat to within a range of 35°C to 40°C, with a maximum

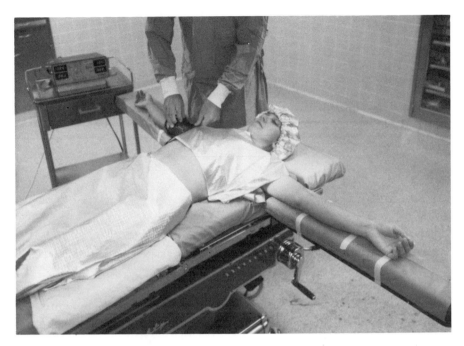

FIG. 5. Thermal barrier drapes and head cover in use as a patient is prepared for surgery. (Courtesy OR Concepts, Inc.)

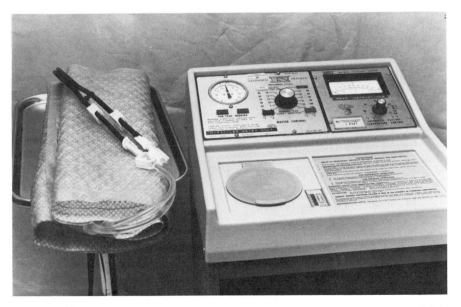

FIG. 6. Heating-cooling system ("hyperthermia, hypothermia unit"). Controller (**right**) folded pad, not connected to controller (**left**).

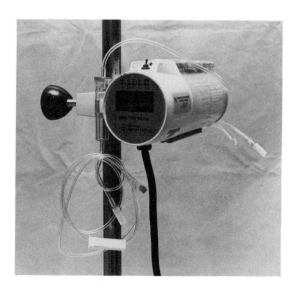

FIG. 7. Dry-heat type fluid warmer with disposable cuff installed. Display at end indicates temperature of warmer.

of 40°C to 42°C. The speed of infusion effects the heating capability of a warmer: if the speed at which fluid passes through a warmer increases, the warmer must work harder to heat the fluid. Most warmers perform well at flows of 50 to 100 ml/minute, but may not be able to maintain the same energy transfer at deliveries of 150 ml/minute.

Virtually all warmers have visual or audio alarms to indicate they have passed a preset maximum temperature, and most incorporate a gauge or dial to indicate heater temperature. Note that the fluid loses heat after leaving the warmer and before entering the patient; ideally, the fluid temperature should be monitored and regulated where it enters the patient, rather than at the warmer. Warmers should reach operating temperature in 5 to 7 minutes, and temperature should not vary by more than 3°C as the warmer cycles. As with other equipment in the OR, warmers should have hospital grade power cords and plugs, be electrically safe, and not be affected by electromagnetic interference from nearby surgical devices.

Fluid warmers should not present excessively hot surfaces. They are especially subject to spills of fluid that may find their way into the electrical components of the device and create an electrical hazard. Spills of blood or plasma on the warm surfaces provide an ideal site for bacterial growth. Therefore, particular attention should be paid to careful inspection and cleaning of fluid warmers as soon as possible after use.

It is worthy of note that a third approach to warming fluids, that of microwave radiation, has been attempted and quickly abandoned. Microwaves provide heat by vibrating molecules rapidly, and the use of this technology seemed to eliminate all the problems of in-line warming methods. One manufacturer produced a dedicated "microwave blood warmer" in the 1960s. Unfortunately, microwave radiation may heat unevenly depending on the material and temperature of the object, and localized underheating and overheating results. In the case of whole blood, overheating and the consequent damage to blood components is a significant risk to the patient. Nonprotein IV solutions may be warmed by some anesthesiologists in this way, but careful attention must be paid to temperature in each case.

ELECTROENCEPHALOGRAPHY (EEG)

The central role of anesthesiologists is to provide patients a safe anesthetic with minimal compromise of organ function. To assess the level of compromise, the clinicians may monitor as many as ten variables; most of these have traditionally been some aspect of cardiovascular or respiratory function. Until the 1970s, little attention was paid to objective measurements of brain function; measures of cerebral activity were limited to pupilary dilation and presence of a gag reflex. Yet the anesthetic catastrophes most feared have always included irreversible losses of brain function. One speaker on this topic stated that most medicolegal catastrophes involve the brain. Since the 1970s increased study and electronic design have generated several models of cerebral function monitors with the surgical environment in mind. These systems are intended to detect dangerous events during surgery, such as seizure activity or localized lack of blood perfusion to the brain, or to enable the physician to regulate drug dosages for maximum benefit but minimum brain depression. These devices are to indicate the depth of anesthesia, although there is some debate here.

The brain, like certain other tissues in the body, generates electrical activity. Its millions of neurons collectively create voltages in the range of 500 microvolts (mV) at the brain surface, or about 50 uV when detected at the scalp. These signals are seemingly random waves which vary in frequency from near 1 Hz to as high as 100 Hz; the average, however, is about 10 Hz depending on brain activity. (Compare this with the average frequency of the ECG at about 1.5 Hz.) EEG signals with a frequency between 0 and 40 Hz usually are considered to be in the normal range.

"Raw" EEG waveforms generally are not used by anesthesiologists as a brain monitor during surgery (Fig. 8). Excessive time away from patients would be required to abstract the frequency range and strength of the waveforms, as well as a substantial amount of equipment and support. In order to compress the raw EEG into information useful to the anesthesiologist, computer-based equipment was developed that ana-

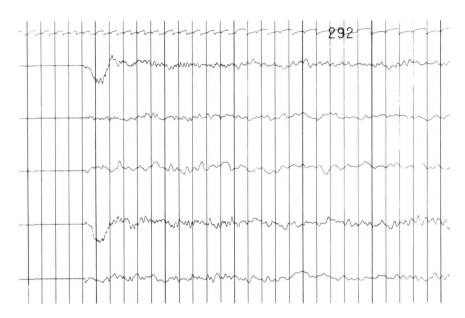

FIG. 8. Typical five-channel recording of "raw" EEG. Paper speed = 30 mm/sec. Complete diagnostic EEGs have sixteen channels.

lyzes and displays the EEG signals in terms of frequency and power at regular intervals (or "epochs"), separately for the right and left sides of the brain. The electronics sample the waveform at many instantaneous points in each epoch, then perform a mathematical operation (Fast Fourier Analysis, FFA) which determines the amount of power at each of many frequencies (Fig. 9). The system also determines that frequency below which 97% of the power exists in each epoch, and indicates it on the display; this "spectral edge frequency" is considered to be a useful trending reference for depth of anesthesia.

Three or four models of interoperative computerized EEG monitors are currently available. They are similar in the methods used to acquire and process the signal, but differ widely in their means of displaying the resultant data. Most use five surface electrodes; usually a recording electrode is attached above each eye and behind each ear, and a ground electrode is placed midline on the forehead (Fig. 10). One unit offers three different display formats: raw EEG from the right and left sides of the brain; a bar graph of the power in various frequency bands; or a "compressed spectral array" (CSA) which presents the power versus frequency traces taken at each epoch over the past 2 to 20 minutes (Fig. 11). Another EEG monitor portrays the information as a pair of 3-dimensional rectangles of frequency versus power versus time, using colors to denote frequency bands (Fig. 12). Still another monitor displays an over-

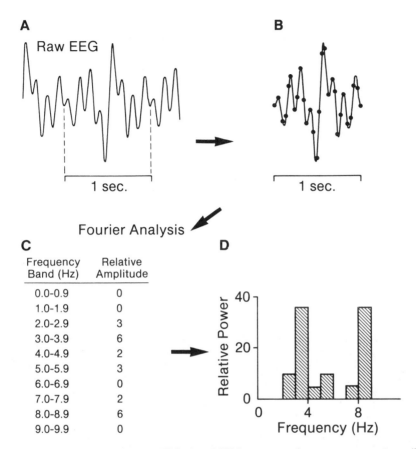

FIG. 9. Illustration of how raw EEG signal (**A**) is converted to a power spectrum (**D**). Dots superimposed on one sec of raw EEG (**B**) show points sampled by the electronics for Fast Fourier Analysis (FFA). Numerical results of FFA are shown (**C**) and graphic display is shown (**D**). (Reprinted with permission from Levy, et al. (1980): *Anesthesiology* Lippincott, Philadelphia, PA.)

view of the head, using sixteen circles (eight on each side) of varying size and color to indicate power and frequency range respectively (Fig. 13). All of these monitors have some means of denoting the spectral edge frequency for each epoch, and most provide a means by which to record their output information for later study.

Because an EEG monitor detects and amplifies such small voltages, the meticulous application of EEG electrodes is critical to its successful operation. The electrodes are identical to, but smaller than, those used for ECG recordings. The patient's skin must be carefully prepared before attaching each electrode. Surface oil is removed by use of a mild solvent, then the contact site is vigorously rubbed to remove the superficial layer

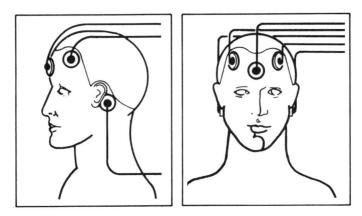

FIG. 10. Typical location of five EEG electrodes for anesthesia brain monitors. (Courtesy Neurometrics, Inc., San Diego, CA.)

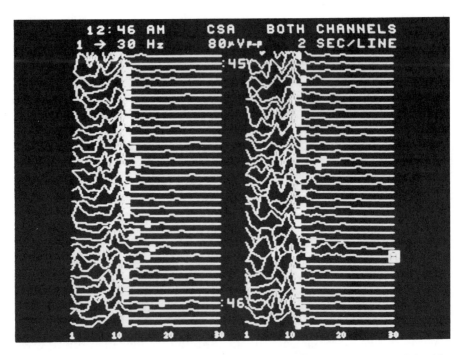

FIG. 11. Compressed spectral array of EEG recorded from the left and the right side of the brain. (Courtesy Interspec Corporation, San Diego, CA.)

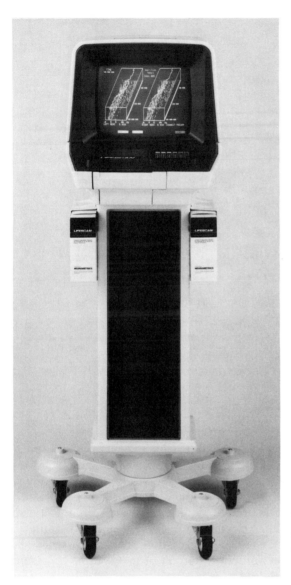

FIG. 12. Processed EEG in each hemisphere displayed in "glass boxes." Continuous white line in each denotes the spectral edge frequency. (Courtesy Neurometrics Corporation, San Diego, CA.)

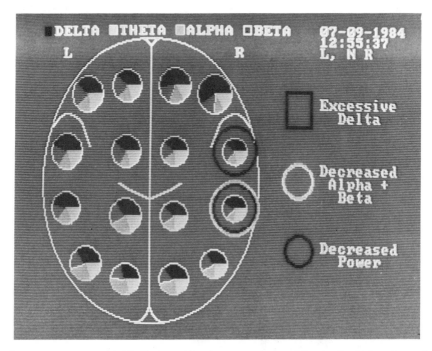

FIG. 13. Processed EEG displayed in sixteen regions of the brain. Colors in each region denote proportions of activity in each frequency band. (Courtesy CNS, Inc., San Diego, CA.)

of dry skin. Application kits are available which include all the electrodes, solvent swabs, an abrasive gel, and gauze. After the electrodes are attached, the wires which connect the electrodes to the monitor should be secured out of the way of personnel and moving equipment; cable motion can be a major source of signal noise. Interference is also possible from skeletal muscle, eye movement, ECG, and electrocautery. The electronics can filter out many of these EEG artifacts, but not all. Most monitors have a connection check circuit or test routine to assure adequate signal before proceeding.

Most EEG monitors have optional circuitry which enables monitoring of the brain's response to a controlled periodic stimulus elsewhere on the body. This *evoked potential* can provide a reference for the competence of the central nervous system during surgeries, especially those which threaten the spinal cord or cerebrum. Instrumentation and technique for recording evoked potentials are not discussed in this book. In some institutions, an EEG technician assists with evoked potential recordings and with EEG recordings.

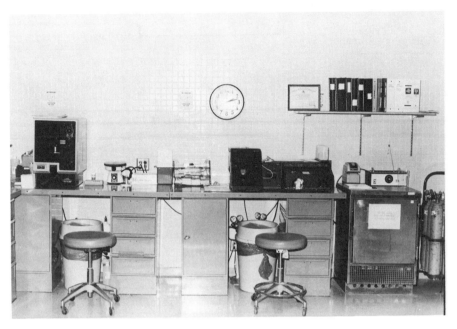

FIG. 14. Photograph of STAT Lab work bench. SOP's and equipment manuals are on shelf (**upper right**).

STAT LAB

Anesthesiologists may request laboratory tests during the course of an anesthetic and expect rapid reporting (within minutes) of results so any remedial action required can be instituted. The most common test requested may be the arterial blood gas analysis. Other tests commonly requested include: serum Na, K, and Cl, and ionized calcium. At some institutions the laboratory tests are done by the clinical pathology department. At other institutions, some tests are done by clinical pathology and some are done in an OR stat lab; or, at some institutions all tests are done in an OR stat lab. Administrative control over the labs also varies from lab to lab. Furthermore, some laboratories participate in a certification program. We will describe in some detail how laboratory tests are processed at our institution.

Within the OR suite is a laboratory which is certified as a Special Functions Laboratory by the College of American Pathologists (CAP) (Fig. 14). Certification applies only to blood gas analysis. Also available is equipment to do serum electrolytes, ionized calcium, COP, and oxygen saturation. CAP certification is an ongoing process; initial certification requires extensive documentation of standard operating procedures

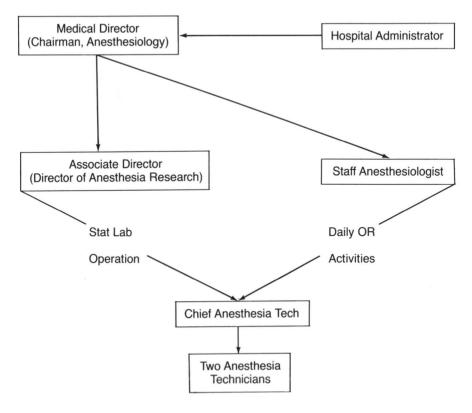

FIG. 15. Organization chart for STAT Lab at Texas Tech University Health Sciences Center and Lubbock General Hospital, Lubbock, Texas.

(SOP's), a documented and rigid quality control program, and a clearly defined organizational structure (Fig. 15).

The Chairman of the Department of Anesthesiology is the Medical Director of the laboratory; the Director of Anesthesia Research is the Associate Director; and the Chief Anesthesia Technician is responsible for the day-to-day operation of the lab. A staff anesthesiologist in the operating room directly supervises the daily activity of the technicians; only anesthesia techs are certified to do blood gas analysis.

The hospital buys equipment needed for the lab and pays for supplies and maintenance; it also pays the anesthesia techs' salaries. In turn, the hospital collects the fee charged for the tests.

SOP's for the equipment, as well as the equipment operation manual, are kept by the instrument. The SOP specifies maintenance requirements and how to do calibration checks. A log of calibration checks is maintained as is a log of when maintenance is performed. The periodical maintenance varies from daily to monthly. The chief anesthesia tech reviews these logs, initials them, and indicates the date of review. Then the Associate Director or Medical Director reviews the logs, approximately every three months, and initials and dates them.

Every three months, coded ampules (surveys) are received from the College of American Pathologists for PO_2, PCO_2, and pH determination. Results are returned to CAP where they are pooled with results from all other participating laboratories. Then the results are returned to the laboratory giving the laboratory's results, and how they compare with results from other laboratories.

The laboratory is inspected annually. One year the laboratory does a self-inspection, the next year CAP does the inspection. CAP provides a self-inspection form which is completed and mailed to CAP. The self-inspection involves the following: the Chief Anesthesia Tech completes the CAP inspection form, the Associate Director reviews the completed form, and an experienced inspector from the Pathology Department does an inspection.

Chapter 9

Medical Gases

MEDICAL GASES AND CYLINDERS

Gases used during the course of anesthesia include oxygen and nitrous oxide; and less frequently, carbon dioxide, air, and helium. These chemicals must be supplied in the compressed state so a continuous supply for a practical period of time is available. In the compressed state, a gas can be supplied in practical quantities from any of several different sizes of cylinders, giving the advantage of portability and the disadvantage of limited volumes (Fig. 1). In the compressed, liquid state, some gases (e.g., O_2) can be supplied from bulk storage tanks at great advantages in capacity and cost, with the obvious disadvantage that the gas must be piped throughout a building and made available at carefully placed outlets in walls and ceilings.

The standards for the construction and periodic testing of all gas cylinders are set and enforced by the U.S. Department of Transportation (DOT), as that agency is concerned with the safe transport of any potentially hazardous containers and materials. Additionally, the National Fire Protection Association (NFPA) and the Compressed Gas Association (CGA) set standards in this country for the labeling, storage, and deployment of cylinder gases. The actual purity of gases for medical use is specified in the United States Pharmacopeia (USP) and enforced by the Food and Drug Administration (FDA). The USP requires 99% purity for virtually all gases prepared for clinical use.

By DOT standards, all medical gas cylinders must bear a series of markings (stamped, not labeled) denoting the type of metal used in the manufacture of the cylinder, the service pressure (i.e., that maximum pressure at which it is charged for customer use), a serial number, and markings for both the manufacturer and the owner of the cylinder. (The vast majority of cylinders remain the property of the gas supplier, and the hospital or clinic using the gases pays a small fee for each use of the cylinder.) Additionally, the cylinder markings show the date of the last testing of the cylinder and an identifying mark for the testing facility (Fig. 2). All cylinders must be tested every 5 years by subjecting them

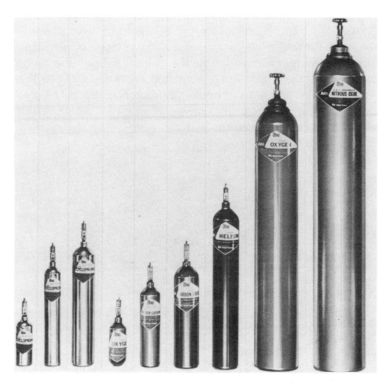

FIG. 1. Nine different sizes of medical gas cylinder. (Courtesy Air Products and Chemicals, Inc., Allentown, PA.)

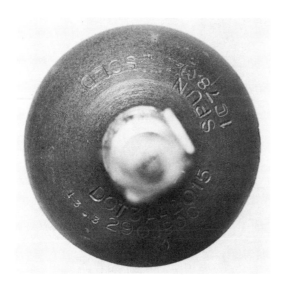

FIG. 2. Stamped cylinder markings required by DOT on an E cylinder.

to at least 1.66 times their normal service pressure without leaks or failure. Routine visual inspections should be made by user as well as supplier to check for leaks, corrosion, and any evidence of physical impact or distortion. In any case of doubt, the cylinder should be taken out of service, labeled as unsafe, and returned to the supplier. While the stamped markings attest to cylinder competence, the CGA requires a distinctive diamond-shaped label on every cylinder which specifies the gas contents, its fully-charged pressure at room temperature, and appropriate warnings about the use of the gas (Fig. 3).

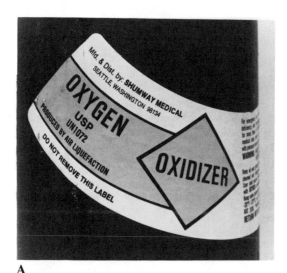

A

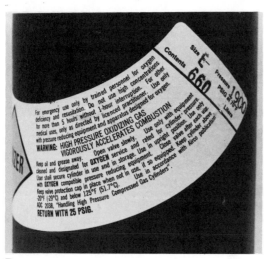

B

FIG. 3. A,B. Typical labeling of an oxygen E cylinder.

The physical dimensions and volumes of the most commonly used medical gas cylinders and the capacities, pressures, and color coding for the five most commonly used gases are seen in Table 1. E cylinders containing oxygen or nitrous oxide are frequently used in clinical settings; the G variety is usually used for larger supplies of those gases. D cylinders are used for limited supplies of gases where size and weight considerations are important. Note that the volume of gas in a cylinder varies, depending upon the gas; this is because of the physical properties unique to each gas. However, oxygen and air are similar and therefore, the volumes of air and oxygen in full cylinders of the same size are virtually identical; the same is true for carbon dioxide and nitrous oxide. For each gas, there is a fixed fill pressure regardless of cylinder size, again determined by the characteristics of the gas. CO_2 and N_2O are in the liquid state in cylinders but exit from them in the gas state. Because of this conversion, the cylinder pressure (e.g., 745 psi for N_2O) remains constant as long as there is any liquid in the cylinder (Fig. 4). When the last few milliliters of liquid escape, the pressure quickly drops to zero. The cylinder pressure gauge reading for these two common medical gases, therefore, is not a useful indicator of the amount of gas remaining. Any significant drop in the gauge reading indicates that the cylinder is very near depletion and that it should be replaced. This is in contrast to all other common medical gases which are in the gas state in the cylinder; cylinder pressure falls gradually as the gas is used. As a practical rule, it is wise to replace an oxygen or air cylinder when its gauge pressure falls to 500 psi.

The hazards of transposing cylinders were obvious long ago, and reports document many disastrous results due to confused gas supplies. In the mid-1950s, the British set a color-coding standard for medical gases in order to minimize this threat. This standard has almost become international, but the U.S. has not yet fully adopted it (see Table 1). The notable exceptions to the international code in the U.S. include oxygen and air. This should be kept in mind if dealing with equipment originating from countries other than the U.S. The color coding extends, logically, to the color of the hoses, connectors, knobs, and gauges on medical equipment.

The preparation of oxygen by the supplier involves a process of "fractional distillation." Air (a mixture of oxygen and nitrogen) is liquefied by compressing it. Then it is carefully decompressed to a pressure at which nitrogen "boils-off" and oxygen remains in the liquid state. Minor impurities left in the liquid oxygen are removed, and the product is transferred to bulk storage tanks, or converted to a gas for cylinder storage.

Nitrous oxide is commercially prepared by heating ammonium nitrate (NH_4NO_3) in two stages. At about 190°C, the chemical fuses; then, with the assistance of a catalyst and heating to 230°C, it converts to nitrous

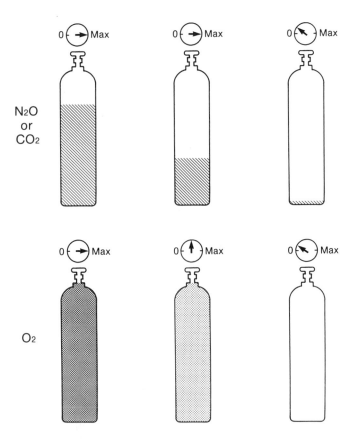

FIG. 4. Comparison of gauge readings of gas supplies which remain as liquids (N_2O or CO_2, **above**) with those which are entirely gaseous at room temperature. Gauge indication of O_2 (or air) will drop gradually as the gas is drawn; that of N_2O or CO_2 will remain at cylinder maximum until the last portion of liquid converts to gas. (Reprinted with permission from J. A. Dorsch and S. E. Dorsch (1984): *Understanding Anesthesia Equipment,* 2nd ed. Williams & Wilkins, Co., Baltimore.)

oxide and water. After purifying by fractional distillation, it is usable as the medical grade product. Medical grade air is not in fact atmospheric air; it is "reconstituted." Producers can produce a medically pure product more economically by mixing pure oxygen and nitrogen in the proportions of 21% and 79% than they can by filtering out the small quantities of trace gases from atmospheric air.

Cylinders of medical gases must be treated with respect. Each one represents a tremendous amount of energy waiting to be released; if released too quickly, that energy can, and has, caused disastrous results. Oxygen and nitrous oxide will support combustion, and so present a fur-

TABLE 1. *Specifications for most commonly used medical gas cylinders*

Dimensions[a]	Cylinder			Color code	
	D	E	G	Int'l.	U.S.
Diameter	11.4	11.4	24.1		
Length	43.2	66.0	129.5		
Volume[b] and Pressure[c]					
AIR: v	405	662	7,356	Black	Yellow
p	2,015	2,015	2,492	& White	
CO_2: v	946	2,590	16,086	Gray	Gray
p	838	838	838		
He: v	365	496	6,79L	Brown	Brown
p	2,015	2,015	2,492		
N_2O: v	946	1,590	15,899	Blue	Blue
p	745	745	745		
O_2: v	405	659	5,570	White	Green
p	2,015	2,015	2,492		

[a]Dimensions in cm
[b]Volume in liters, at room temperature
[c]Pressure in pounds/in^2
Source: Handbook of Compressed Gases, 2nd ed. Compressed Gas Association, New York, 1981.

ther safety problem. The following guidelines from the CGA and NFPA should be adhered to consistently:

1. Cylinders must be kept in an area which is cool, clean, and well-ventilated.
2. Full cylinders should be stored separate from empty ones (Fig. 5).
3. A cylinder should always be secured in a rack, support, or chain, or connected to its utilizing device. If a small cylinder must be unsecured temporarily, keep it out of foot traffic.
4. Before putting a cylinder into service, it should be inspected for labeling and physical defects; all wrappings and dust should be cleared away.
5. A fresh sealing washer should always be in place before attaching a small cylinder to a regulator or machine (Fig. 6).
6. Before connecting a new cylinder to a regulator or machine, it is considered good practice to "crack" it (i.e., remove its protective cap or seal and *slowly* open the valve just enough to allow gas to clear the exit port of any dust or debris).
7. After attachment to a regulator or machine, the cylinder valve should be opened *slowly* using a wrench intended for the purpose, and the valve should be opened *fully* (counter-clockwise until it stops). A cyl-

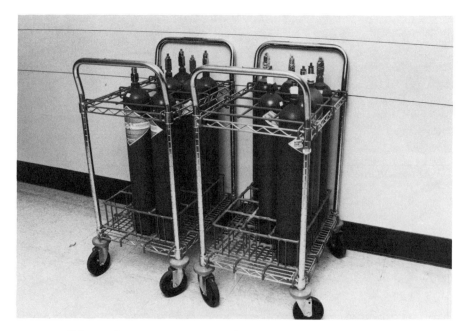

FIG. 5. Separate storage racks for full and empty gas cylinders.

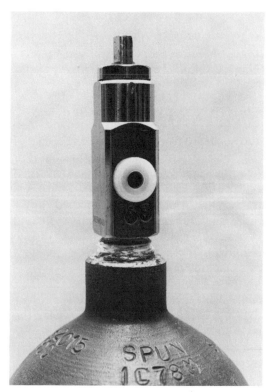

FIG. 6. Plastic sealing washer provided on the smaller sizes of cylinder. When tightened onto a yoke or regulator, the washer compresses and prohibits any gas leakage.

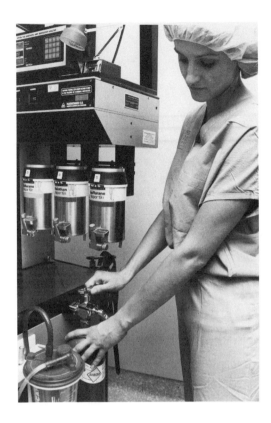

FIG. 7. Securing and opening a cylinder to an anesthesia machine.

inder valve is not a pressure regulator; it is either fully open or fully closed. Keep head and face away from the exit port of the valve when opening (Fig. 7).

8. When the cylinder is empty, or if suspected of being close to empty, it should be taken out of service and replaced.
9. *Never,* under any circumstances, alter or obscure the labeling or coloring of a cylinder, or attempt to alter or disassemble a valve or regulator.

GAS CONNECTION INDEXING SYSTEMS

Pin Indexing for Small Cylinders

By the early 1950s, it was obvious that there was an ever-present danger of attaching the wrong gas cylinder to a machine, thereby delivering dangerous, if not lethal, gas mixtures to a patient. Anesthesia personnel, then without the benefit of monitors routinely used today, could unknowingly administer 100% nitrous oxide instead of 100% oxygen. To elimi-

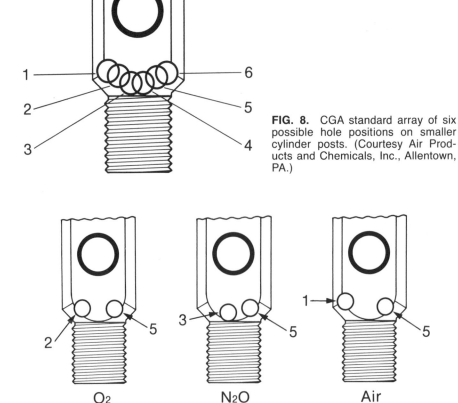

FIG. 8. CGA standard array of six possible hole positions on smaller cylinder posts. (Courtesy Air Products and Chemicals, Inc., Allentown, PA.)

FIG. 9. CGA standard for pin hole positions of three common medical gases. (Courtesy Air Products and Chemicals, Inc., Allentown, PA.)

nate this risk, a pin indexing system was established by the CGA for cylinder sizes A through E. The standard specifies positions in an arc below the outlet port; for any gas or gas mixture, only 2 of these holes are drilled (Fig. 8). On the anesthesia machine yoke, or on any regulator, are ⅛″ diameter pins in the corresponding positions. Thus, a cylinder can only be connected to a yoke or regulator for which it is intended. Substitution of a cylinder of any other gas is not possible as the pins will not allow the post to mate and seal with the yoke (Fig. 9).

No attempt should ever be made to defeat the purpose of this system by filing or removing the pins on a yoke or regulator assembly. After years of use, the pins on a device may loosen or fall out, in which case the device should be repaired or discarded (Fig. 10).

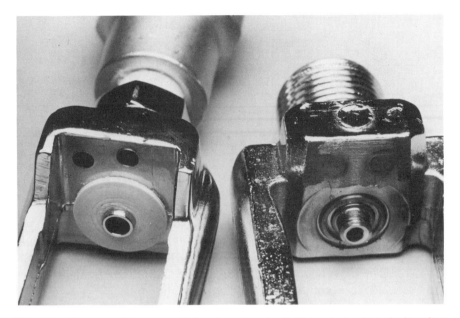

FIG. 10. Two potential causes of disasters: air yoke (**left**) is missing its indexing pins; pins for O_2 yoke (**right**) have been sawed off.

Valve Connector Indexing for Large Cylinders

While the same risk of misconnections exists with large cylinders, it is impractical to use a pin-indexing system for them. Instead, each gas is indexed to a specific threaded connector at the cylinder outlet. The connectors vary according to thread orientation (internal versus external or "female" versus "male"), thread polarity (right-hand versus left-hand), diameter, and the design of the nipple which seats in the connector (Fig. 11). Thus, it is impossible to connect a regulator or manifold intended for nitrous oxide to an oxygen cylinder. The various connector combinations are specified by a CGA standard and designated by a three-digit number.

Wall Outlet and Hose Connector Indexing

As hospital and clinic building design evolved in the 1950s and 1960s, piped supplies of oxygen, nitrous oxide, air, and vacuum became standard. The advantages in terms of safety, economy, and convenience were obvious. But the interface between these utilities and the utilizing devices presented the same possibilities for misconnection that cylinders had. Again, the CGA set a standard for a system of mating threaded

Valve Assembly

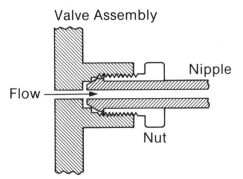

Flow

Nipple

Nut

FIG. 11. Diagram of outlet connector for large gas cylinders. Thread polarity and nipple diameters are specific to each type of gas. (Reprinted with permission from J. A. Dorsch, and S. E. Dorsch (1984): *Understanding Anesthesia Equipment*, 2nd ed. Williams & Wilkins, Co., Baltimore.)

connectors which are specific to only one gas. The variable in each connector type is the diameter of the nipple side and its mating bore on the body; thus, it is referred to as the Diameter Index Safety System (DISS) (Fig. 12). The CGA added an additional series, after the original standard was defined, to accommodate the metric system and newer gas combinations; but lack of interchangeability remains the essential feature. The convention in equipment design is that the male-threaded body component of the connector is available at wall outlets, ceiling manifolds, and at the utilizing device (ventilator, anesthesia machine, etc.); and the nipple-and-nut assembly is provided on each end of the hose between source and device (Fig. 13).

After the DISS standard was introduced, several manufacturers marketed their own gas-specific connector sets, with the added feature that they utilize the line gas pressure to enable the rapid disconnection of devices, with minimal manipulation and without the use of tools (Figs. 14A,B). Generically referred to as "quick connects," these connector sets have generally had widespread acceptance in medical facilities, especially in the operating room; but, depending on design and materials, some have shown a greater failure rate than others. Users should be observant for loose indexing pins and failing spring action on these connectors. Equally important, the choice of quick-connects system for devices in a hospital should be made in concert with all departments responsible for those devices; incompatibility between a device connector and the supply connectors in various patient care areas can be a direct threat to patient safety. Adapter assemblies are available when it is necessary to connect dissimilar connector types (Fig. 15).

The design of gas supply hoses is also specified in a standard. Hoses and connectors are engineered for a maximum of 200 psi, even though the conventional delivery pressure is 50 psi. Hoses have a 0.25 inch inside diameter and 0.46 inch outside diameter, use an imbedded braid in the wall for added strength, and should be color-coded around the full

Body   Nipple and Nut Assembly

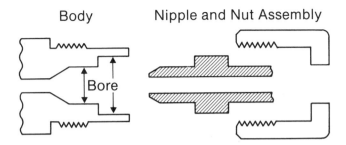

FIG. 12. Diagram of Diameter Index Safety System (DISS) connector. Diameters of the larger and smaller bores are specific to each type of gas. (Reprinted with permission from J. A. Dorsch, and S. E. Dorsch (1984): *Understanding Anesthesia Equipment,* 2nd ed. Williams & Wilkins, Co., Baltimore.)

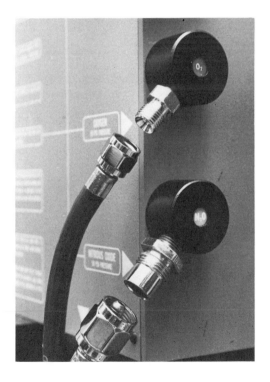

FIG. 13. DISS connectors for O_2 and N_2O at an anesthesia machine.

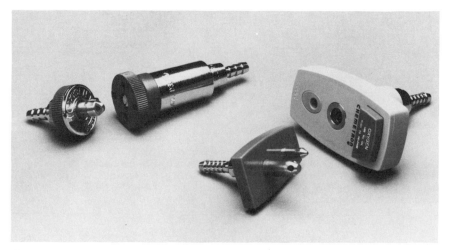

A

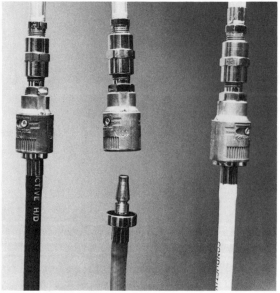

B

FIG. 14. A,B. "Quick connect" type gas connectors.

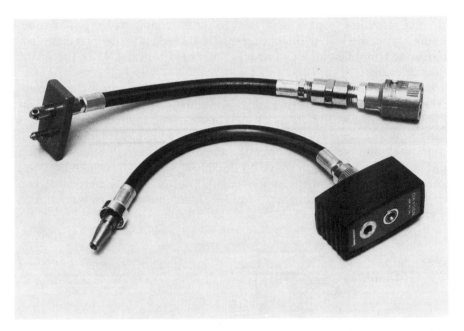

FIG. 15. Adapter assemblies, which are necessary to connect devices to gas supplies with dissimilar connector types.

circumference for a specific gas. Earlier types had a thinner wall and a single, less easily seen, color-coding stripe. After years of use, hoses can weaken, swell, or crack. Health care personnel should be observant for these failures and have the hoses repaired or, preferably, replaced.

REGULATORS

Anesthesia requires the delivery of gases to the patient in flows of up to 10 L/min., with occasional need for "flushing flows" of 40 to 70 L/min. Obviously, the very high pressures at the outlet of a supply cylinder must be reduced so that flows can be safely and conveniently maintained. Anesthesia machines are designed to accept supply pressures of 50 psi; therefore, the 2,000 psi within an E cylinder of O_2 and 745 psi in a N_2O cylinder must be greatly reduced. This is accomplished by a regulator which consists of two chambers in a common housing, with a small opening between them. Two springs are arranged in balanced opposition to each other to control a valve between the two chambers. In the "direct acting" type, the valve is opened slightly by adjusting the main spring tension so it is greater than that of the sealing spring, thereby offsetting the balance between the two. This, in turn, allows a portion of the high pressure to pass from inlet-to-outlet chamber. In the "indirect acting" type, the high cylinder pressure is allowed into the inlet chamber, and passes into the outlet chamber at the reduction valve when the spring balance is upset (Fig. 16).

Both types of regulator depend on a balance between high pressure exerted over a small area (the valve seat), and low pressure exerted over a large area (the outlet chamber membrane). The indirect acting type is more prevalent in modern equipment, as it is inherently safer. All regulators include a vent port above the membrane on the outlet chamber, and must include a safety valve on the outlet side to allow high pressure to escape in the event of component failure. Many machines use two stages of regulation in the interest of safety and to minimize fluctuations

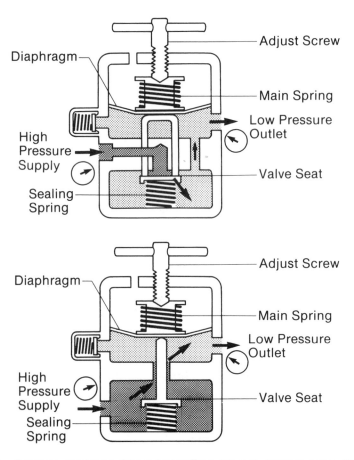

FIG. 16. Pressure regulators. Direct-Acting Type (**above**). Indirect-Acting Type (**below**). (Reprinted with permission from J. A. Dorsch, and S. E. Dorsch (1984): *Understanding Anesthesia Equipment,* 2nd ed. Williams & Wilkins, Co., Baltimore.)

in flow due to fluctuations in supply pressure. Regulators on anesthesia machines are preset at the factory for the conventional 50 psi (Fig. 17). They should never be tampered with and require no maintenance. The most likely failure of a regulator is at the membrane, but failures are quite rare. Occasionally, particulate contamination can be trapped in the valve seats, causing them to behave erratically, or allowing the high-pressure supply to pass through. In either case, the unit should be taken out of service for repair by qualified personnel.

Supply gas is led from the reduction valve to a flow control valve. A flow control valve essentially is a needle valve on a finely-threaded stem; the pin or needle seats in a conical port (Fig. 18). Turning the knob gradually unseats the needle, allowing increasing gas flow. Most flow control valve knobs have stops which prevent the user from overtightening the closed valve, thereby bending or even breaking the needle. Flow valves should always operate smoothly, any stiffness or abrupt flow changes may indicate a dirty or defective valve, which should be serviced.

In the earliest anesthesia machines, flow was indicated by a small push rod within a calibrated glass tube; gas flow forced the rod up within the tube. The need for greater accuracy at lower flows brought the use of the Thorpe tube, in which the rod is replaced by a floating ball or bobbin

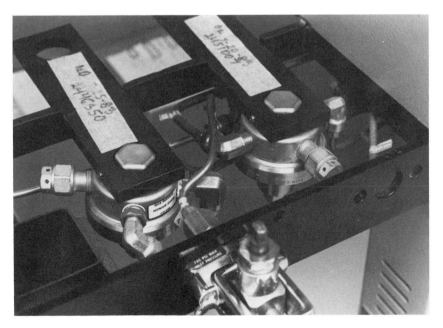

FIG. 17. Regulators for N_2O **(left)** and O_2 **(right)** on an anesthesia machine. Factory-set outlet pressure is adjusted at a hex nut; note the escape vents protruding from body of each regulator.

Seat

Stem

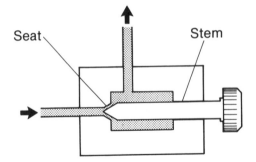

FIG. 18. Flow control valve. (Reprinted with permission from J. A. Dorsch, and S. E. Dorsch (1984): *Understanding Anesthesia Equipment,* 2nd ed. Williams & Wilkins, Co., Baltimore.)

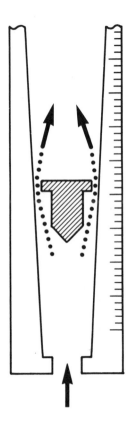

FIG. 19. Flow indicator tube and bobbin. Calibrations on tube may or may not be linear. (Reprinted with permission from C. Petty (1987): *The Anesthesia Machine.* 1st ed. Churchill-Livingstone, New York.)

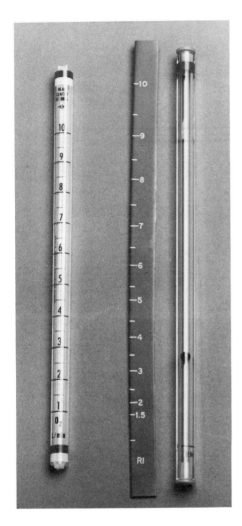

FIG. 20. Flow tube for two different anesthesia machines. Tube with integral calibrations (**left**). Tube and calibration board, to be mounted together (**right**).

(Fig. 19). The float often has markings and flutes which cause it to rotate within the tube, serving as a visual indication that it is floating free and is not stuck. The inside diameter of the clear tube has a gradual taper so that the upper diameter is greater. This enables the tube to be calibrated for low flows (200 to 1,000 ml/min) near the tubes' bottom, and higher flows (up to 10 L/min) at top. Flowmeters are factory calibrated as a set: tube, float, and calibration board (Fig. 20). The flow through the set is determined by the properties of the gas, the inside diameter of the tube, the mass of the float, and to a lesser degree, the ambient temperature and pressure.

PIPELINE GAS SUPPLIES AND VACUUM

The piped supplies of gases and vacuum commonly found in hospitals and clinics are essential to safe patient care. Their construction and maintenance are invariably the responsibility of the building engineering department, but any employee who uses these utilities should have a basic understanding of them. Oxygen and suction (vacuum) are essential in every patient care location. Nitrous oxide is usually supplied to any location where anesthesia is administered: the OR, the delivery room, ambulatory surgeries, and in specialty areas such as Lithotriptor units, laser procedure rooms, and radiology. Piped air is also a useful adjunct to anesthetic practice, especially in pediatrics, and so is found in the OR as well as in areas where respiratory therapy is administered. High-pressure nitrogen is the ideal gas for driving many surgical tools and is piped into the OR in larger or newer facilities.

Oxygen

Bulk oxygen supplies are those with a capacity of more than 20,000 cubic feet of gaseous oxygen. In medium and large medical facilities, oxygen is stored as a liquid in a large tank which is essentially a thermos bottle (Fig. 21). To keep oxygen in its liquid state at $-183°C$, the tank wall is multi-layered with insulation and a near-vacuum exists so that little heat energy transfers from the outside to vaporize the liquid. A small amount of vaporization is unavoidable, but the gaseous oxygen produced internally can be released into the atmosphere by a relief valve. Liquid is converted to gas for user demand via a vaporizing device which supplies just enough heat to the liquid to maintain adequate gas pressure. The vaporizer consists of a coil, tube, or mesh situated at the tank which is heated by electricity or hot water. Gauges indicate liquid level and pressure in the tank. One cubic foot of the liquid converts to 860 cubic feet (24,347 liters) of gas at room temperature and pressure. Gaseous oxygen from the vaporizer is drawn-off and heated in order to obtain the desired line pressure, and a regulator downstream maintains pressure $\pm$ 10%. Liquid oxygen supplies are delivered by tank trucks.

A pressure monitoring device constantly assures that the gas pressure to the building remains $\pm$ 10% of the intended value. If the pressure increases or, more likely, decreases beyond that range, an alarm sounds at strategically placed locations and the reserve supply is brought online. Because of the complexity of the piping systems in larger institutions, the primary supply pressure may be as high as 75 psi, which is reduced to 50 psi at branches to user areas. At specific points downstream, there are branch shut-off valves (Fig. 22). All health care workers should be aware of the location of these shut-offs, line pressure gauges, and alarm

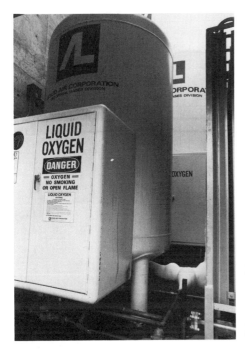

FIG. 21. Bulk oxygen supply tanks for a medium-sized medical center. Primary tank (**back**); secondary (**front**). Box (**left**) contains gauges and valves for pressure regulation. Note frost accumulation on delivery pipes due to heat exchange as cold O_2 gas warms to ambient temperatures.

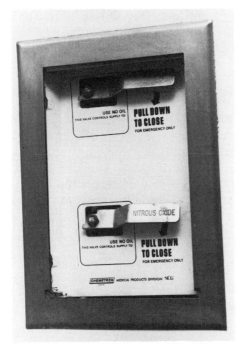

FIG. 22. Branch supply shut-off valves for O_2 and N_2O.

terminals (Fig. 23). Under no circumstances, however, should the shut-off valves be tampered with unless users have specific authorization, and then only after assuring that user personnel are notified. NFPA standards require that bulk oxygen supplies are supported by a reserve supply, which can be brought into service in the event of any failure of the primary supply. This may be a second, smaller liquid system or a number of large cylinders (G or H) connected to a common manifold and regulator (Fig. 24).

Nitrous Oxide

Nitrous oxide, although a liquid under moderate pressure, is not usually supplied from a single bulk supply tank as is oxygen. It remains practical to use a dual battery or bank of G or H cylinders for a hospital pipeline supply (Fig. 25). Each bank of four to six cylinders is connected to a manifold with its own shut-off valve and regulator; both banks are connected with a common pressure-sensitive switch and an alarm. Only one bank is in use at any given time; when that bank begins to deplete, the pressure monitor detects a drop in pressure and automatically switches on the alternate bank. The nitrous oxide supply is often kept in a remote location of the building, frequently the basement. In the process of vaporizing from its liquid state, nitrous oxide draws heat from the surrounding cylinder, manifold, and regulator; so much so that it is common to see frost formation on these components (Fig. 26). If the location of the supply is subject to cold ambient temperatures, it is possible for the regulator to freeze and fail.

Air

Compressed medical air in institutional pipeline systems is almost universally supplied from the ambient atmosphere, not from USP-grade cylinder air. Typically, a pair of large air compressors draw air from an elevated point of the building through a series of filters, and fill a holding tank of sufficient capacity to allow for the typical demands of the various departments (Fig. 27). Regulators assure that the line pressure remains at 50 psi ± 10%, and the compressors automatically turn on to resupply the holding tank when the demand reduces the supply pressure below 45 psi. Pipeline compressed air is not "reconstituted" as is cylinder medical air; it is filtered at the entry point and again downstream from the holding tank. The NFPA sets allowable limits for impurities in these systems, notably for: carbon dioxide, carbon monoxide, hydrocarbons, particulates, and water. Water can be an expensive problem in air supplies: as it always exists in the atmosphere and is compressed in the supply, water

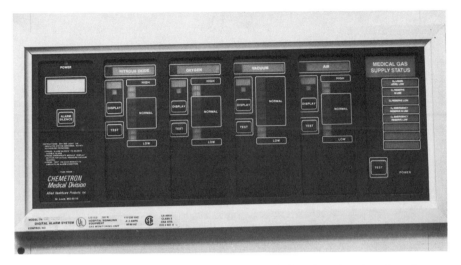

FIG. 23. Gas pressure alarm panel in a hospital engineering department.

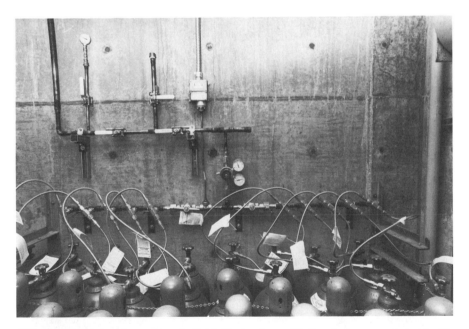

FIG. 24. Reserve O_2 supply manifold. Photo shows 20 G cylinders connected to 10 points on the manifold; half are switched on-line at a time. Small tube (**center**) of manifold connects to gas alarm switch on wall. Reserve supply should enable 8 hours of typical demand.

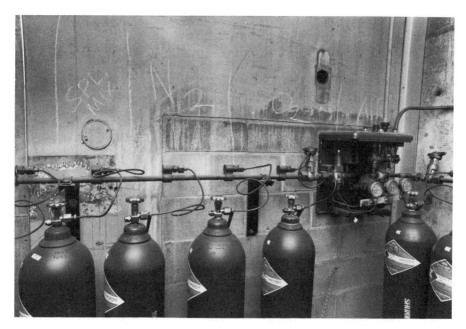

FIG. 25.   Nitrous oxide supply bank. One set of 4 cylinders is on-line at a time. Switchover and alarm sensor are in corner **(right)**.

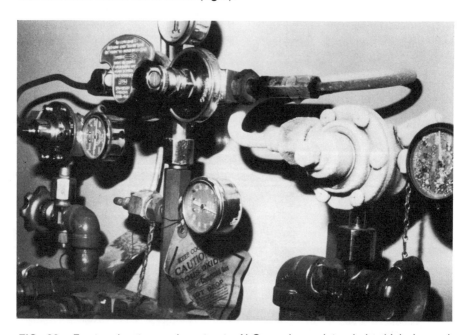

FIG. 26.   Frost and water condensate at a N_2O supply regulator during high demand period.

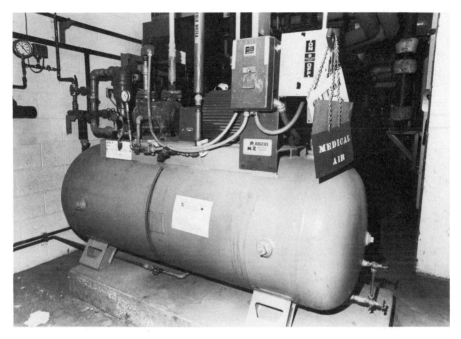

FIG. 27. Medical air supply compressors and holding tank. Delivery pipe and gauge can be seen on wall (**left**).

vapor will "rain-out" throughout the system. If not removed by heater-traps at various branches of the supply, it can cause serious damage to patient care devices. Medical personnel should be alert for evidence of moisture at air outlet connectors or within anesthesia equipment, ventilators, and air-oxygen blenders.

Vacuum

Vacuum systems are critical in life-threatening patient care procedures. Adequate suction is essential when significant amounts of fluid must be aspirated from a patient's upper airway or chest, or from a traumatic or surgical wound. The vacuum system is also used to remove noxious or hazardous fumes from the pharmacy, clinical pathology laboratory, and operating room. In most facilities, a large capacity suction pump is the source of vacuum for the entire building, often backed-up by a second on-call pump (Fig. 28). Traps are put in vacuum systems to prevent fluids or particulates from being drawn into the pump. The primary safeguard for the system is a trap at *every* user connection. *Never* use a vacuum outlet without a trap or "collection jar." This may be a glass or, more commonly, disposable plastic receptacle with capacities

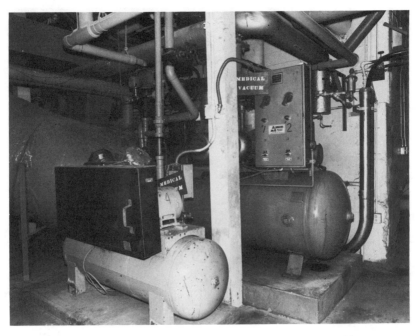

FIG. 28. Two medical vacuum sources of different capacities.

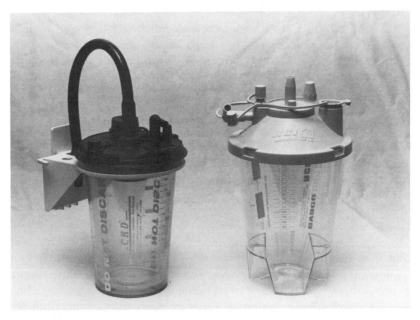

FIG. 29. Examples of disposable suction traps. Model using a disposable liner (**left**); unit that is totally disposable (**right**). Site where vacuum is connected and where suction hose is connected is marked on the trap.

from 1 L to 4 L. Configuration of receptacles vary according to manufacturer, but all models are constructed so that where the vacuum is applied is above where the fluid enters (Fig. 29). If the container fills to
near capacity, a valve will close the vacuum supply port.

Vacuum is measured in inches of mercury column height (Hg). As the
nominal pressure of the atmosphere at sea level is 29.9 Hg (or 760
mmHg), a "perfect" vacuum would be -29.9 Hg (expressed without the
minus sign). Engineering standards for medical vacuum systems require
at least 15 Hg at a flow of 30 L/min.

Chapter 10

Drugs Used in Anesthesia

In this section, we will introduce the generic names of drugs used in anesthesia and identify how they are packaged for use. The pharmacology of these agents is discussed in a variety of texts (e.g., Gilman, Goodman, Rall and Murad, PDR), and will not be discussed in detail here. Given the nature of anesthesia practice, the anesthesiologist may administer any drug currently available. This discussion is limited to those drugs most frequently used in most institutions by anesthesiologists.

It is important to know that drugs have at least three names: a chemical name, a generic name, and one or more trade names (Appendix 1). The chemical name is derived from the chemical structure of the drug molecule, using standard nomenclature; the generic name is one recognized by an official body (the US Adopted Names Council); and the trade name is the registered name for the drug formulation marketed by a drug company. In the clinical setting, it is preferable to use the generic name.

A usual sequence of drug administration for routine elective surgeries where the patient is given a general or local anesthetic is shown in Appendix 2. A list of drugs commonly used by anesthesiologists and the purpose for which they are used is seen in Appendix 2.

Common intraoperative drugs would include analgesics, amnesics, muscle relaxants, agents to increase or decrease blood pressure, and drugs to adjust blood pH. While used infrequently, dantrolene is kept available to treat or prevent malignant hyperpyrexia, a syndrome triggered by some drugs (e.g., certain inhalation anesthetics and neuromuscular blocking agents).

With the exception of the inhalation agents, the drugs are supplied in ampules, vials, or syringes, and are administered via needle and syringe. The drug usually is in liquid or crystal form. In the latter case, the crystals are dissolved in liquid (vehicle) before injection. The vehicle may be aqueous (e.g., local anesthetic) or organic (e.g., diazepam). The organic solutions generally are "thicker" (more viscous) than are the aqueous solutions and therefore are more difficult to draw into and eject from a syringe.

Combining aqueous and organic solutions generally is not recom-

APPENDIX 1. *Different names for a local anesthetic*

Chemical	Generic
dl-1-butyl-2′ 6′ pipecoloxylidide	bupivacaine

Trade
Marcaine® (Winthrop-Breon) Sensorcaine® (Astra)

APPENDIX 2. *Usual sequence of drug administrations for general or regional anesthesia*

General Anesthesia	Regional Anesthesia
Premedication Intravenous induction agent Neuromuscular blocking agent Inhalation and/or intravenous anesthetic/analgesic Neuromuscular blocking agent antagonist	Premedication Local anesthetic agent

APPENDIX 3. *Drugs commonly used by anesthesiologists*

Premedicants

Analgesics: morphine, meperidine
Anxiolytic: diazepam, midazolam, lorazepam
Reduce salivation and prevent heart rate decrease: atropine, scopolamine
Reduce gastric secretion and/or motility: cimetadine, metoclopromide
Prophylaxis of aspiration pneumonitis: sodium citrate, sodium citrate with citric
   acid
Anesthetic induction agents: thiopental, etomidate, ketamine, propofol
Inhalation anesthetic agents: halothane, isoflurane, enflurane, nitrous oxide
   (N_2O)
Injectable anesthetics/analgesics used usually in conjunction with other agents to
   maintain anesthesia: fentanyl, sufentanil
Neuromuscular blocking agents: curare (dtc), vecuronium, atracurium,
   pancuronium, succinylcholine
Agents to adjust blood pH: sodium bicarbonate
Agents to reduce blood pressure: sodium nitroprusside, trimethaphan,
   propranolol, labetalol, clonidine, verapamil, nifedipine
Agents to increase blood pressure: calcium chloride, calcium gluconate,
   epinephrine, dopamine, isoproterenol, dobutamine
Local anesthetic agents: procaine, chloroprocaine, lidocaine, mepivacaine,
   tetracaine, bupivacaine, prilocaine
Opioid antagonists: naloxone
Reversal of neuromuscular blocking agents: edrophonium, pyridostigmine,
   neostigmine
Agents to treat cardiac arrhythmias: lidocaine, verapamil, bretylium

mended as a cloudy solution will be formed. For the same reason, solutions with different pH generally should not be mixed (e.g., lidocaine. HCl pH 6.6, thiopental Na pH 10.5). At some institutions, the pharmacy prepares all drug solutions, including any mixing and placing into syringes.

Ampules are opened by breaking off the top. A file for scoring the ampule at the intended break point is sometimes supplied. One should use gauze sponges to grip the ampule when breaking off the top to reduce the chance of cutting oneself. Contents of vials usually are accessed via needle penetration of a rubber diaphragm which seals the top of the vial.

Read the label of the container to be sure that the container contains the drug desired, the concentration of the drug is the desired concentration, and the form of the drug is the form desired (e.g., lidocaine. HCl versus lidocaine CO_2; lidocaine. HCl with epinephrine). All loaded syringes must be labeled, indicating syringe contents (drug/solution, concentration, date). There is now a color-coding standard for these labels (ASTM D10.34).

The inhalation agents are bottled in liquid form in 125 or 250 ml amber glass containers (halothane, isoflurane, enflurane) or in gas cylinders (N_2O). The inhalation agent is placed in a vaporizer on the anesthetic machine for delivery. N_2O exits the cylinder in gaseous form. Its flow to the patient is controlled by flowmeters on the anesthetic machine.

Chapter 11

Bibliography

1. *Textbook of Advanced Cardiac Life Support.* (1987): American Heart Association, Dallas, Texas.
2. American National Standard for Anesthetic Equipment-Tracheal Tubes. ANSI 279:14-1983. American National Standards Institute, 1430 Broadway, New York, NY 10018.
3. American Society of Anesthesiology. The Anesthesia Care Team. Park Ridge, Illinois.
4. Bilt, C. D. (ed). (1985): *Monitoring in Anesthesia and Critical Care Medicine.* Churchill Livingstone, New York.
5. *Biomedical Safety and Standards Newsletter.* Quest Publishing. Brea, CA.
6. Bowie, E., and Huffman, L. (1985): *The Anesthesia Machine: Essentials for Understanding.* Ohmeda Corp., Madison, WI.
7. Brown, B. R. (1984): *Future Anesthesia Delivery Systems: Contemporary Anesthesia Practice.* F. A. Davis Co., Philadelphia, PA.
8. Carr, J. J., and Brown, J. M. (1981): *Introduction to Biomedical Equipment Technology.* John Wiley and Sons, Inc., New York.
9. Characteristics and Safe Handling of Medical Gases (1987): Pamphlet P-2. Compressed Gas Association, New York.
10. DeMarre, D. A., et al. (1979): *Applied Biomedical Electronics for Technicians.* Dekker, New York.
11. Dorsch, J. A., and Dorsch, S. E. (1984): *Understanding Anesthesia Equipment,* 2nd ed. Williams & Wilkins, Baltimore.
12. Gravenstein, J. S., and Paulus, D. A. (eds) (1982): *Monitoring Practice in Clinical Anesthesia.* J. B. Lippincott, Philadelphia, PA.
13. *Health Devices* (monthly). ECRI. Plymouth Meeting, PA.
14. *Health Devices Alerts* (semi-monthly). ECRI. Plymouth Meeting, PA.
15. Hill, D. W. (1972): *Physics Applied to Anaesthesia.* Appleton-Century-Crofts, New York.
16. Kirby, R. R., Smith, R. A., and Desautels, D. A. (1985): *Mechanical Ventilation.* Churchill Livingstone, New York.
17. Klein, S. L. (1985): *A Glossary of Anesthesia and Related Terminology.* Medical Examination Publishers Co., Inc., New Hyde Park, New York.
18. Martin, J. T. (ed). (1987): *Positioning in Anesthesia and Surgery,* 2nd ed. W. B. Saunders Co., Philadelphia, PA.
19. May, S., et al. (1985): *Capnography in the Operating Room. An Introductory Directory.* Raven Press, New York.
20. McMahon, D. J., and Thompson, G. E. (1987): *A Survey of Anesthesia Support Personnel in Teaching Programs.* Med. Inst., 21: 269.
21. *Medical Instrumentation* (bi-monthly). Association for Advancement of Medical Instrumentation. Arlington, VA.
22. Miller, R. D. (ed). (1986): *Anesthesia.* Vols. 1-3. Churchill Livingstone, New York.
23. Minimum Performance and Safety Requirements for Components and Systems of Continuous-Flow Anesthesia Machines; #F-29 (1987): American Society for Testing Materials, Washington, D.C.

24. Mogue, L. R., and Rantala, B. (1988): Capnometers. *J. Clin. Monit.* 4:115-121.
25. Mushin, W. W., and Jones, P. L. (1987): *Macintosh, Mushin & Epstein: Physics for the Anaesthetist*, 4th ed. Blackwell Scientific Publications, Boston.
26. Petty, C. (1987): *The Anesthesia Machine*. Churchill Livingstone, New York.
27. Schreiber, P. (1972): *Anaesthesia Equipment*. Springer-Verlag, Berlin.
28. Schreiber, P. (1984): *Safety Guidelines: Anesthesia Systems*. N. A. Drager, Telford, PA.
29. Schreiber, P. (1985): *Anesthesia Systems*. N. A. Drager, Telford, PA.
30. Smith, J. J., and Kampine, J. P. (1984): *Circulatory Physiology: The Essentials*. Williams and Wilkins, Baltimore, MD.
31. Spooner, R. B. (1980): *Hospital Electrical Safety Simplified*. Instrument Society of America, Research Triangle Park, N.C.
32. Standard for Safety: Medical and Dental Equipment; #UL 544 (1987): Underwriters Laboratories, Park Ridge, IL.
33. Webster, J. G. (ed). (1978): *Medical Instrumentation*. Houghton-Mifflin, Boston.

Subject Index